EMT EMERGENCY MEDICAL TECHNICIAN

CRASH COURSE®

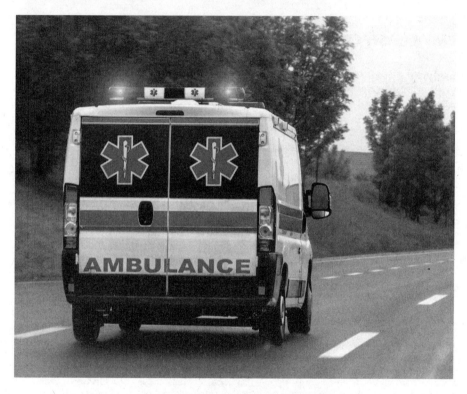

Chris Coughlin, PhD, NRP, NEMSEC

Research & Education Association
www.rea.com

ABOUT REA

Founded in 1959, Research & Education Association (REA) is dedicated to publishing the finest and most effective educational materials—including study guides and test preps—for students of all ages.

Today, REA's wide-ranging catalog is a leading resource for students, teachers, and other professionals. Visit *www.rea.com* to see our complete catalog.

Research & Education Association
1325 Franklin Ave., Suite 250
Garden City, NY 11530
Publisher email: info@rea.com
Author email: ccoughlin@contracosta.edu

EMT CRASH COURSE,® 3RD EDITION

Printed in the United States of America

Library of Congress Control Number 2023915843

ISBN-13: 978-0-7386-1287-4
ISBN-10: 0-7386-1287-1

Cover image: © iStockphoto.com/OgnjenO
Author photo (back cover) by Joey Gutierrez

REA Crash Course® and REA® are trademarks of Research & Education Association.

EMT CRASH COURSE
TABLE OF CONTENTS

PART I

Introduction

PART II

Preparing to Become an EMT
Review plus end-of-chapter practice

PART III — Assessment, Airway, Respiration, and Ventilation
Review plus end-of-chapter practice

PART IV — Pharmacology, Cardiology, and Resuscitation/Stroke
Review plus end-of-chapter practice

PART V — Shock, Trauma, and Environmental Emergencies
Review plus end-of-chapter practice

PART VI — Medical, Obstetrics, and Gynecology
Review plus end-of-chapter practice

PART VII

EMS Operations
Review plus end-of-chapter practice

PART VIII

After the Exam

Online Glossary........................ available at *www.rea.com/EMT*
Online Practice Exam... available at *www.rea.com/studycenter*

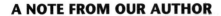

A NOTE FROM OUR AUTHOR

You are one test away from making life-or-death decisions in potentially dangerous circumstances. It is not practical to try and learn everything in your EMT textbook. If it's important, it's probably in the textbook; however, not everything in the textbook should be memorized in preparation for the national certification exam. The advantage of this fully updated *EMT Crash Course* study guide is that it emphasizes the must-know content.

That said, this *Crash Course* is not a substitute for a well-written textbook, nor does it take the place of participating in a high-quality EMS training program. Rather, this book is a bridge between your training and your NREMT exam. The book focuses on information in three specific areas:

1. How to stay safe as you serve your community as an EMS professional.

2. How to ensure you are a competent EMS professional.

3. How you should prepare for the national certification exam.

Experience is a tough teacher. In EMT class, you received the lessons first and then took the tests. When you respond to 9-1-1 calls as an EMS professional, the tests come first, without warning, and the lessons follow. When you are not prepared for class, you risk a poor grade. When you are not prepared for the street, people can get hurt. Study hard. Stay safe. Don't lose focus on the rewarding career that is just around the corner for you.

Regards,

Chris Coughlin

ABOUT OUR BOOK

REA's *EMT Crash Course* is designed for the last-minute studier or any EMT candidate who wants a quick refresher before taking the NREMT Certification Exam. This *Crash Course* will show you how to study efficiently and strategically, so you can pass your exam.

Written by a veteran EMS Program Director, NREMT paramedic, and nationally certified EMS educator, REA's *EMT Crash Course* gives you a review specifically targeted to what you really need to know to pass the exam.

- **Parts I and II** get you started with tips for succeeding on the exam, along with an overview of the EMT's role and responsibility within the larger public health system, as well as a survey of the anatomy of the human body.

- **Parts III, IV, and V** cover the components of the EMS System including patient assessment, resuscitation and AED, trauma, medical and environmental emergencies, pharmacology, as well as evidence-based guidelines for delivering patient care.

- **Part VI** explains special patient care, with particular attention to pediatric and geriatric patients.

- **Part VII** reviews EMS operations, such as ambulance and air medical operations, mass casualty incidents, and weapons of mass destruction.

- **Part VIII** looks ahead to what you should do after you pass your exam.

- **End-of-chapter practice questions** help you review what you've learned.

- An extensive **medical glossary** with more than 400 study terms is available for download at *www.rea.com/emt*.

ABOUT OUR PRACTICE EXAM

Are you ready for the NREMT exam? Find out by taking **REA's online practice exam** available at *www.rea.com/emt*. Your performance is automatically scored and comes with detailed explanations for every answer. Use this valuable study tool to pinpoint your strengths and weaknesses so you'll be ready on exam day.

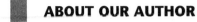

ABOUT OUR AUTHOR

Dr. Chris Coughlin is Emergency Medical Services Assistant Professor and Paramedic Studies Program Director at Contra Costa College in San Pablo, California. Dr. Coughlin is a nationally certified EMS instructor. In 2006, he became one of the first 850 nationally certified flight paramedics (FP-C) in the United States. He previously worked as a critical care flight paramedic in Phoenix, and served as the Department Chair of Public Safety Sciences at Glendale Community College in Glendale, Arizona. He is also the author of REA's *Paramedic Crash Course*.

Dr. Coughlin has degrees in Paramedicine from Glendale Community College, Adult Education from Ottawa University, and Educational Leadership from Northern Arizona University. He holds a doctorate in Educational Philosophy from Capella University.

Dr. Coughlin welcomes correspondence at ccoughlin@contracosta.edu.

AUTHOR'S DEDICATION AND ACKNOWLEDGMENTS

Dedicated to...

My children: Saren Coughlin, RN; Hannah Coughlin, RN; Alissa Coughlin, RN; and Nathan Coughlin, Cognitive Assessment Specialist.

My wife, Lisa Coughlin, Senior Application Developer. *Tu sei il mio mondo!*

Thank you to...

Aaron Bates
EMT Program Director
Contra Costa College

Rainier Perez
EMS Program Director
Glendale Community College

Special thanks to all the dedicated EMTs that serve their communities every day (and night!). Thank you for enduring the long hours, sleepless nights, move-ups, postings, late calls, and immense stress of serving others on their worst day. They call and you come, any time, every time. Thank you!

PUBLISHER'S ACKNOWLEDGMENTS

Publisher: Pamela Weston

Editorial Director: Larry B. Kling

Technical Editors: Aaron Bates (book), Rainier Perez (online practice test)

Copy Editor: Fiona Hallowell

Digital Content Prep: Heidi Gagnon

Book File Prep: Jennifer Calhoun

Typesetting: Caragraphics

PART I

INTRODUCTION

Preparing for Success on the National Certification Exam

Becoming a nationally certified Emergency Medical Technician (NREMT) lets the public, employers, and state licensing authorities know that you have demonstrated competency. The exam is rigorous, comprehensive, and highly effective at assessing entry-level competency. This book is intended to help ensure that when you submit your answer to that last question on the exam, you become (for a short time), the newest NREMT in the United States. Let's get to work!

This chapter is designed to do three things:

1. Demystify the exam. If you know what to expect, you can better prepare.

2. Provide information and tips that will help you prepare and reduce your stress level about the exam.

3. Identify the essential content you need to know to pass the test.

I. THE EXAM

The National Registry EMT exam is a "pass/fail" test. Its purpose is to identify who is competent. Your future patients don't care what you scored on the exam; however, they do care about getting competent and compassionate care for themselves and those they care about.

The exam is a computer-adaptive test (CAT). The sophisticated software driving the exam adapts to your individual abilities. This means everyone will feel like the test was challenging. The exam delivers one question at a time, and the questions are **not** randomly chosen. With each answer you submit, the software is honing and updating its estimate of your ability level. The estimate gets more precise as the exam progresses. The exam ends when there is 95% certainty that your competency level is either above or below the passing standard.

The NREMT exam complies with the Americans with Disabilities Act (ADA) by offering reasonable accommodations for individuals with disabilities.

II. TOPICS COVERED ON THE EXAM

The exam covers five broad content areas. You will likely answer at least 70 and no more than 120 questions. You will have two hours to complete the exam. The exam was developed with input from over 3,500 content experts. Questions on the exam are anchored in the National EMS Scope of Practice Model, the National EMS Education Standards, and the National Registry Practice Analysis.

NREMT Exam Topics	% of Test by Topic
Airway and ventilation	18%–22%
Cardiology, resuscitation, stroke	20%–24%
Trauma	14%–18%
Medical and OB-GYN	27%–31%
EMS operations	10%–14%

Source: https://www.nremt.org/Document/cognitive-exams

For all but EMS operations, 85% of the questions relate to adult patients and 15% relate to pediatric patients. Although not separate categories, topics such as patient assessment, anatomy & physiology, pediatric emergencies, and safety are emphasized throughout the test.

Author's Note: You can find more information on the format of the exam at *nremt.org/document/cognitive-exams*

III. QUESTION FORMATS

The NREMT has expanded the types of questions you will encounter on National Registry certification exams. Although there will be plenty of traditional multiple-choice questions on your exam, it will also include so-called technology-enhanced items (TEIs) that deploy computer technology to better simulate clinical practice.

One type of TEI you're likely to see is called a multiple-response item. Unlike traditional multiple-choice questions, multiple-response items contain more than once correct answer option. Such items are weighted the same as other questions on the exam and no partial credit is given.

Multiple-response item Example 1:

Which of the following are directional terms? Select the TWO answer options that apply.

    A. north

    B. dog

    C. left

    D. biscuit

    E. purple

Options A and C are correct. Both options must be selected to be considered correct.

Multiple-response item Example 2:

Which of the following are traffic signs? Select the THREE answer options that apply.

    A.

    B.

    C.

    D.

    E.

    F.

Options A, C, and E are correct. All three options must be selected for your answer to be considered correct.

The four additional question formats you may see include Build List, Sequencing, Drag-and-Drop, and Check Box. Here's how these item types will be presented:

Build List   You are given a list of options on the left side of a split screen. You are then tasked with following a set of instructions to organize the list in the answer area on the right side of the screen.

Example: "Organize the following from most to least concerning."

Sequencing   You are provided a set of answer choices that must be sorted into a specific order.

Example: "Place the following actions in the proper order."

Drag-and-Drop   You select and reposition answers from a list or graphic.

Example: "Place the following therapies in the correct list as either indicated or contraindicated."

Check Box   You respond with a checkbox feature, like a survey response.

Example: "Click the box to indicate your response."

By adding TEIs to the certification exam, the National Registry seeks to make the test-taking experience more engaging and reflective of conditions in the EMS field. For additional information about question types on the NREMT exam, including further examples, visit *www.nremt.org/Document/TEIs*.

IV. SCORING

Typically, you can retrieve your exam results from the NREMT website within two business days by logging into your account. You will *not* be given your score or be able to review your test. If you do not pass the exam, the NREMT will provide information about your performance on each of the five exam categories. Candidates must wait at least 14 days before scheduling another attempt. Of course, this doesn't apply to you because *you're going to pass!*

V. PREPARATION

What does solid preparation for the NREMT certification exam entail? Read this book! That is the first, but not only, step to get ready to do your best. Most people only retain what they read for a short time. To help absorb what you read, apply an active learning format that works for you. Examples of active learning activities include the following:

- Flashcards
- Mental imagery
- Verbally reciting content
- Writing exercises
- Highlighting key information for review
- Practice questions
- Study groups
- Having someone quiz you

VI. GENERAL TEST-TAKING TIPS & STRATEGIES

- Take the test as soon as you can after completing your EMT course. We forget information we aren't using frighteningly fast. The chances of passing go down steadily over time.
- Study every day! Don't cram or procrastinate.
- CPR! Prepare for every conceivable CPR-related question you can think of. The CPR questions on the exam are based on the current American Heart Association Guidelines for CPR and Emergency Cardiovascular Care.
- You don't need to read this book in the order it is presented. If you like, go directly to the content you think requires the most attention.
- Be well-rested before taking the test. Avoid caffeine, energy drinks, excess sugar, etc., right before the test. These will not improve your performance or steady your nerves.
- Know exactly where the testing center is and arrive early. Bring the required identification.
- Dress comfortably. Bring a sweater if you get cold easily.

VII. DURING THE TEST

- Take a moment to quiet your mind and focus on your breathing. Believe in yourself.

- The test will have a clock telling you how much time is left.

- You will have access to an on-screen version of the Texas Instruments TI-108 Elementary Calculator.

- You **cannot** skip a question or return to it later.

- Read the entire question and each answer choice thoroughly. There is usually something specific in the question that points you toward the correct answer.

- Irrelevant information is eliminated from the question stem during the review process by NREMT. Bear in mind that all the information in the question is included for a reason. Don't add anything to the question or make a "what-if" scenario from it.

- In most cases, you'll be dealing with standard multiple-choice items. This means only one response option is correct, and you will likely be able to eliminate two of the answer choices quickly. At first blush, the remaining answer choices may both seem correct, but—in a question with just one correct answer—one must be better than the other. Count on something in the question pointing you toward the better choice. Find it.

- When in doubt, *treat*. Recall your priorities during patient assessment, especially during the primary assessment. This will help with many of the scenario-based questions.

- Relax! The test is going to feel hard. This does **not** mean you are failing.

 VIII. ADDITIONAL INFORMATION

For additional information and updates about the certification exam, visit the NREMT website at *https://www.nremt.org/Document/cognitive-exams*.

PART II

PREPARING TO BECOME AN EMT

History, Public Health, and the EMT's Role

I. TERMS TO KNOW

A. **9-8-8:** National Suicide & Crisis Lifeline.

B. **Emergency medical dispatcher (EMD):** A dispatcher specially trained to give medical instructions to 9-1-1 callers.

C. **Enhanced 9-1-1:** Automatically ties a location to the call—either with a street address or geographic coordinates.

D. **Medical director:** The physician responsible for providing medical oversight in a healthcare facility.

E. **Quality improvement (QI):** Continuous review and auditing of all aspects of the EMS system to identify areas of improvement.

II. THE EMERGENCY MEDICAL SERVICES (EMS) SYSTEM

A. EMS is a coordinated network of personnel and resources designed to provide care and transportation of patients to the appropriate higher level of care.

B. EMS is also part of the larger public health system and participates in public education and prevention efforts.

III. HISTORY OF THE EMS SYSTEM

A. EMS is still a young profession compared to other healthcare professions, such as nursing.

B. The modern EMS system evolved from battlefield medicine, ambulances operated by funeral homes, and volunteers. The quality of prehospital care varied greatly until the 1970s.

C. The 1960s

1. In 1966, a paper titled "Accidental Death and Disability: The Neglected Disease of Modern Society" is published by the National Academy of Sciences. This document is widely known as the EMS "White Paper."

2. The White Paper is regarded as heralding the beginning of modern EMS. It spotlights inadequacies of prehospital care in the U.S., particularly related to trauma.

D. The 1970s

1. The U.S. Department of Transportation (DOT) develops the first EMT National Standard Curriculum (NSC).

2. The first EMT textbook is published.

3. Later in the decade, the DOT publishes the first paramedic NSC.

E. The 1980s

1. The American Heart Association (AHA) dramatically increases its emphasis on heart disease prevention, science, and education.

2. Additional levels of training are added to the existing EMT and paramedic curricula.

3. Broad differences remain in the scope of practice for certification levels from state to state.

F. The 1990s

1. The National Registry of EMTs (NREMT) advocates for a unified national training curriculum.

2. The National Highway Traffic Safety Administration (NHTSA) begins work on the *EMS Agenda for the Future.*

3. Public access defibrillation sweeps across the U.S. and significantly changes survival rates for out-of-hospital cardiac arrest.

G. The 2000s

1. The first National EMS Education Standards (NEMSES) are developed, replacing the previous National Standards Curricula.

2. Four new levels of national EMS certification are developed:

   i. Emergency Medical Responder

   ii. Emergency Medical Technician

      iii. Advanced Emergency Medical Technician

      iv. Paramedic

H. Major additions to NEMSES for EMTs:

    1. Administration of beta agonist medications

    2. Administration of anticholinergic medications

    3. Administration of OTC analgesics

    4. Blood glucose monitoring

    5. CPAP

    6. Pulse oximetry

    7. Assisting higher-level providers

IV. COMPONENTS OF THE EMS SYSTEM

A. Public access: Refers to how the public accesses the EMS system.

B. Clinical care: Outlines the scope of practice and associated equipment.

C. Medical direction: Physician oversight of patient care.

D. Integrated health services: EMS personnel work with hospital personnel to ensure continuity of care.

E. Information systems: The information technology component of EMS.

F. Prevention: The EMS system's role in preventing injury and illness.

G. Research: Moving EMS toward evidence-based care.

H. Communications: Systems used to activate EMS, dispatch responders, and communicate with medical direction.

I. Human resources: Efforts to professionalize the EMS occupations.

J. Legislation and regulation: Ensures EMS conforms to local, state, and federal requirements.

K. Evaluation: The quality improvement component of EMS.

L. Finance: Funding sources of EMS.

M. Public education: Focuses on EMS system's role in the larger public health system.

N. EMS education: Addresses the quality of EMS training.

V. ACCESSING EMS

A. 9-1-1

1. Most 9-1-1 systems today are "enhanced," which allows the dispatcher to automatically identify the phone number and location of the caller.

2. Emergency Medical Dispatchers (EMDs) are specially trained to give medical instructions to 9-1-1 callers.

3. Nearly 75% of homes do not have a landline, according to a 2022 survey by the National Center for Health Statistics. This can make it more difficult to confirm the location of the incident.

Note: The U.S. national 9-8-8 crisis helpline is intended to reduce confrontations with law enforcement.

B. 9-8-8

1. A new national suicide and mental crisis helpline.

2. Connects callers to trained counselors.

3. Most callers get the help they need through the call itself.

4. Established because 9-1-1 is not well-suited to address acute mental health emergencies.

5. Mental health crises usually lead to a law enforcement response. Nearly 25% of fatal police shootings involve people with mental illness. 9-8-8 aims to reduce confrontations with law enforcement.

C. EMS Practice Analysis

1. Most common adult requests for EMS help: trauma, abdominal pain, respiratory distress/arrest, behavioral problems, seizures, and syncope.

2. Highest risk of harm: airway obstruction, respiratory distress/arrest, cardiac arrest, hypovolemic shock, anaphylaxis, stroke, and inhalation injury.

VI. LEVELS OF TRAINING

A. Emergency Medical Responder (NREMR): Provides basic immediate care, such as bleeding control, CPR/AED, epinephrine auto-injector, opioid antagonists, and uncomplicated emergency childbirth.

B. Emergency Medical Technician (NREMT): Includes all EMR skills, advanced oxygen and ventilation skills, pulse oximetry, NIBP monitoring, blood glucose monitoring, and additional medications.

C. Advanced EMT (NRAEMT): Includes all EMT skills, supraglottic advanced airway devices, IV/IO access, and additional medications.

D. Paramedic (NRP): Includes all preceding levels, advanced assessment and management skills, various invasive skills, and extensive medications. This is the highest level of prehospital care outlined in the NEMSES.

Paramedic

AEMT skills plus:
- Needle thoracostomy
- Cricothyrotomy
- Intubation
- PEEP
- ECG interpretation
- Manual defibrillation
- Trans. ext. pacing
- High flow nasal cannula
- Extensive medications

AEMT

EMT skills plus:
- Supraglottic airways
- IV/IO insertion
- Additional meds
- Waveform capnography

EMT

EMR skills plus:
- Nasal airways
- Pulse oximetry
- CPAP
- Auto BP (NIBP)
- Oral OTC analgesics
- Anticholinergic meds
- Blood glucose monitoring
- Mechanical CPR
- Assist in complicated childbirth

EMR

- CPR/AED
- Manual airway
- Oral airways
- BVM
- Oxygen
- Airway suction
- Manual BP
- Epi auto-injector
- Opioid antagonists
- Tourniquets
- Wound packing
- Spinal motion

VII. DESTINATION FACILITIES

A. EMS patients are transported to the appropriate destination based on the chief complaint, patient request, and local protocol.

B. There are several types of specialty facilities, including:

1. Burn centers

2. Stroke centers

3. Cardiac centers

4. Level 1 trauma centers

5. Mental health facilities

6. OB/neonatal centers

7. Pediatric centers

8. Toxicology centers

VIII. EMT ROLES AND RESPONSIBILITIES

A. Equipment preparedness

B. Emergency vehicle operations

C. Scene safety

D. Patient assessment and treatment

E. Lifting and moving

F. Communication and documentation

G. Patient advocacy

H. Professional development

I. Quality improvement

J. Illness and injury prevention

K. Certification and licensure

IX. MEDICAL DIRECTION AND MEDICAL CONTROL

A. Medical director: The physician responsible for providing medical oversight.

B. Medical control: Physician instructions for patient care (direct or indirect). Provided by medical director or designated physician (e.g., base station physician).

   1. Online (direct) medical control: direct contact between physician and EMS provider.

   2. Offline (indirect) medical control: written protocols.

X. PATIENT SAFETY

A. When patients are harmed by EMS providers, it is usually due to poor decision-making, failure to follow established protocols, or failure to perform skills competently.

   1. Preventing errors

      i. Know your protocols and follow them.

      ii. Consult with medical direction.

   2. When in doubt, always do what is best/safest for the patient.

B. Routine activities by EMS providers that are "high risk" for the patient include:

   1. Transfer of patient care: The EMT must provide all necessary information for continuity of care.

   2. Lifting and moving patients: The EMT must avoid injuring the patient during lifting and moving.

   3. Transportation: Occupants in the back of the ambulance are at high risk of injury in the event of a motor vehicle collision.

4. Spinal precautions: Spinal precautions must be taken when indicated. Patients can also suffer if they are placed in spinal precautions when **not** indicated.

5. Medication administration: Medication errors are too common and potentially dangerous.

XI. PROFESSIONAL ATTRIBUTES

A. Professional appearance

B. Skills competency

C. Physical capability

D. Leadership skills

E. High ethical standards

F. Emotional stability

G. Critical and adaptive thinking skills

H. Effective listener

I. Ability to place success of team above self-interest

XII. QUALITY IMPROVEMENT (QI)

A. Also called continuous quality improvement (CQI).

B. Continuous review and auditing of all aspects of the EMS system to identify areas of improvement.

C. Medical director responsible for overseeing the QI process.

XIII. **INTEGRATED PUBLIC HEALTH**

A. EMS is part of the larger public health system.

B. Prehospital care is meant to be integrated with the care delivered at the receiving hospital.

C. Examples include immunization clinics, prevention education, safety & wellness events, public CPR training.

PRACTICE QUESTIONS
Answers on page 379.

1. Which of the following is widely considered to mark the beginning of the modern EMS system?

   A. the EMS White Paper

   B. the current National EMS Education Standards

   C. the creation of the American Heart Association

   D. the EMS Agenda for the Future document

2. Modern EMS care is based on

   A. what has been done in the past.

   B. whatever physicians recommend.

   C. evidence-based medicine.

   D. the original national standard curriculum.

3. Which of the following are professional attributes of the EMT? (Select the TWO answer options that apply.)

   A. always speaking your mind

   B. leadership skills

   C. always taking charge

   D. refusing to transport stable patients

   E. the physical ability to lift and move patients

4. EMT roles and responsibilities include

    A. strong communication skills.

    B. establishing intravenous (IV) access.

    C. swift water rescue.

    D. initial crime scene investigation.

5. Which of the following EMS activities are considered high risk for the patient?

    A. assessing vital signs

    B. obtaining a blood glucose level

    C. requesting consent to treat

    D. transferring patient care

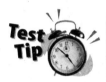

Test Tip

Make a study plan and stick to it. Study a little every day. Don't try to do it all at once and don't procrastinate. Find a place to study that works well for you physically and mentally. Find a study partner or join a study group to hold each other accountable.

Workforce Safety and Wellness/Lifting and Moving/ Patient Restraint

I. TERMS TO KNOW

A. **Bariatrics:** Branch of medicine that deals with the study and treatment of obesity.

B. **Personal protective equipment (PPE):** Equipment and supplies necessary to implement the appropriate precautions for a specific patient encounter.

C. **Resiliency:** The ability to cope with stress without suffering lasting physical or psychological harm.

D. **Standard precautions:** Minimum infection prevention practices that apply to all patient care situations.

E. **Supine hypotensive syndrome:** Hypotension in a pregnant woman who is lying supine.

II. SCENE SAFETY

A. The EMT's first priority is always personal safety. This will never change and is thus a high priority on the certification exam.

B. After personal safety, your priorities are the safety of your partner(s), patient, and bystanders.

C. Maintaining scene safety includes addressing scene-specific hazards, appropriate infection control precautions, safe lifting and moving techniques, safe transport, and appropriate transfer of care procedures.

Note: Scene safety is always the top priority!

III. **EMT WELLNESS**

A. Physical well-being

1. Job tasks require that EMTs maintain a certain level of physical conditioning and get adequate sleep.

2. Sleep deprivation is a known safety issue for EMS providers.

   i. A prolonged period without sleep impairs cognitive function, similar to being intoxicated (20 hours without sleep mimics a legally intoxicated blood alcohol content).

   ii. Many EMS employers with high call volumes no longer allow 24-hour shifts.

3. Address modifiable risk factors for heart disease and stroke.

   i. Don't smoke/vape.

   ii. Manage hypertension and stress.

   iii. Exercise and eat a healthy diet.

   iv. Manage high cholesterol and diabetes.

B. Mental well-being

1. EMTs routinely experience stressful situations, potentially traumatic events, and adverse working conditions.

2. The risk of suicide among EMS providers is much higher than for the general population.

3. Emotional demands of the EMS profession:

   i. Routine exposure to the stages of grief during death and dying:

   ➤ Denial: The patient may experience a "not me" stage.

   ➤ Anger: The patient may experience a "why me?" stage.

   ➤ Bargaining: The patient may experience a "but I still need to . . ." stage.

   ➤ Depression: The patient may experience a state of despair.

   ➤ Acceptance: The patient may come to accept death.

   ii. Routine exposure to high-stress situations, such as:

   ➤ Exposure to violent situations.

➤ Frequent users of the EMS system.

➤ Patients who need more than the EMS system can provide.

➤ Long hours, high call volume, and sleep deprivation.

➤ Aggressive system status management (move-ups, postings).

C. Stress

1. Acute stress: an immediate physiological and psychological reaction to a specific event. The event triggers the body's "fight-or-flight" response.

2. Delayed stress

   i. A stress reaction that develops after a stressful event.

   ii. Delayed stress does not interfere with the EMT's ability to perform during the stressful event.

   iii. Post-traumatic stress disorder (PTSD) is an example of delayed stress.

3. Cumulative stress

   i. The result of exposure to stressful situations over a prolonged period. For many EMTs, this leads to burnout.

   ii. Cumulative stress in EMS providers contributes to anxiety, low job satisfaction, increased clinical errors, ambulance-related accidents, and PTSD.

D. Resiliency

1. Resiliency is the ability to cope with stress without suffering lasting physical or psychological harm.

2. Develop a plan for managing stress.

   i. Recognize signs of stress or burnout:

      ➤ Anxiousness, irritability

      ➤ Headache, poor concentration

      ➤ Loss of appetite, difficulty sleeping

      ➤ Loss of interest in sex, hobbies, work, family, friends

      ➤ Increased use of alcohol, drugs

      ii. Find time for relaxing activities and interests.

      iii. Listen to observations of family and friends. They know you best.

      iv. Balance the demands of your personal and professional life.

      v. Consider a change in your work environment or counseling.

E. Critical Incident Stress Management (CISM)

   1. CISM is a formalized process to help emergency workers deal with stress.

      i. Defusing sessions, when needed, are held within 4 hours of the incident.

      ii. Debriefing sessions are held 24 to 72 hours after the incident.

      iii. CISM teams consist of trained peer counselors and mental health experts.

      iv. CISM is meant to facilitate the process of dealing with critical incident stress. It is not used as a critique of patient care or any other type of performance evaluation.

      v. The information shared during a CISM session is confidential.

IV. INFECTIOUS DISEASE

A. Infectious diseases are caused by an invading pathogen.

   1. Bacterial infections, such as strep throat, usually respond to prescription antibiotics.

   2. Viral infections, such as the flu, are resistant to antibiotics.

   3. Routes of transmission

      i. Diseases can be transmitted from person to person through direct person-to-person contact or indirect contact, such as a doorknob or phone.

      ii. Unlikely objects may be a source of indirect transmission, such as the ambulance driver compartment.

B. Epidemic and pandemic

   1. Epidemic: Widespread occurrence of disease in a community at a particular time.

    2. Pandemic: Outbreak of disease across several countries or continents.

C. Standard precautions

    1. The Occupational Safety and Health Administration (OSHA) oversees regulations concerning workplace safety, including infectious disease precautions.

    2. Employers develop infection control protocols and provide the necessary equipment and training.

    3. Employees are required to complete mandatory training and follow written protocols.

    4. Standard precautions are to be implemented for all patient contacts and are based on the assumption all body fluids pose the risk of infection.

        i. Immediately report exposures to the designated infection control officer.

        ii. Handwashing: This is the single most important way to prevent the spread of infection. Hand sanitizers can be effective, but soap and water are preferred when available.

        iii. Personal Protective Equipment (PPE)

            ➤ PPE is the equipment and supplies necessary to implement the appropriate precautions for a specific patient encounter. PPE can differ from patient to patient based on the exposure risk (bloodborne vs. airborne).

            ➤ Minimum PPE: Gloves and eye protection should be used during any patient contact situation.

            ➤ Expanded PPE

              — Use disposable gown, mask, and face shield for significant contact with any body fluid. For example, childbirth.

              — Use a high efficiency particulate air (HEPA) mask or N-95 respirator for suspected airborne disease exposure, such as tuberculosis.

D. Additional infection control guidelines

    1. Contaminated medical waste should be placed in special "biohazard" bags and disposed of according to local and federal guidelines.

2. Disposable supplies are intended for single patient use. They reduce the risk of exposure and are usually preferred to reusable equipment.

3. Reusable equipment such as stretchers, BP cuffs, etc., must be properly cleaned with an approved disinfectant after every use.

4. "Sharps," such as needles, lancets, etc., are placed in a designated puncture-proof container. Sharps should **not** be recapped before placing in an approved sharps container.

E. Recommended immunizations and vaccinations

1. Regular TB testing

2. Hepatitis B vaccination series

3. Tetanus shot

4. Influenza (flu) vaccine

5. COVID-19 vaccine

6. MMR vaccine: measles, mumps, rubella

7. Varicella vaccine

8. Pneumococcal vaccine

9. Pertussis

V. PREVENTING WORK-RELATED INJURIES

A. Follow your employer's protocols.

B. Use the ambulance's vehicle restraint system properly at all times, including in the patient care compartment during patient transport.

C. Hazardous materials incidents

1. Maintain a safe distance and attempt to keep others out.

2. Call for specially trained hazmat responders.

3. Look for placards without entering the scene and utilize the *Emergency Response Guidebook* (ERG) to determine evacuation distance.

4. Do not begin emergency care until patients have been decontaminated or otherwise cleared by hazmat crews.

D. Crime scenes

1. EMS providers should never enter an active crime scene unless law enforcement has determined it is safe.

2. EMS providers may be advised to respond to the call but maintain a safe distance away until cleared by law enforcement. This is sometimes called "staging for PD."

E. Accident scenes

1. Federal law requires that EMS workers wear an approved highly reflective traffic safety vest when working on roadways, around traffic, or at an accident scene.

2. Use your emergency vehicle to help protect the scene when necessary.

F. Additional hazards requiring specially trained responders

1. Downed power lines, fire situations, etc.

2. Special rescue situations

3. Motor vehicle accidents requiring complex extrication

4. Terrorism incidents

VI. LIFTING AND MOVING

A. Patient safety: Use extreme caution when lifting and moving patients. This is a high-risk activity for both patients and providers.

B. Safe lifting techniques

1. Power lift

   i. Keep object close to the body. Use the legs to lift, not the back (legs bent, back straight).

   ii. Use a power grip with palms up and all fingers wrapped around the object.

2. Position the stretcher to reduce the height of the lift.

3. Preplan the lift to reduce distance and avoid problems.

4. Get enough help.

C. Emergency moves

1. Used when the scene is dangerous and the patient must be moved immediately and before providing patient care.

2. Examples: armpit-forearm drag, shirt drag, blanket drag.

D. Urgent moves

1. Used when the patient has potentially life-threatening injuries or illness and must be moved quickly for evaluation and treatment.

2. Rapid extrication

   i.   An urgent move used for patients in a motor vehicle.

   ii. Requires multiple rescuers and a long backboard.

E. Non-urgent moves

1. Used when there are no hazards and no life-threatening conditions apparent.

2. Examples: direct ground lift, extremity lift, direct carry method, draw sheet method.

F. Log roll technique

1. Commonly used to place a patient on a backboard or assess the posterior.

2. Can be done while maintaining manual cervical spine precautions.

3. Should have at least three trained personnel.

G. Equipment for patient movement

1. Wheeled stretcher

   i.   Secures in the ambulance for transport.

   ii. Usually the safest way to move a patient across smooth, level terrain.

   iii. Most models can accommodate at least 350 pounds.

   iv. Newer models have an automated lift system to further reduce the risk of injury.

2. Portable stretcher

   i.   Lightweight, compact stretcher.

    ii.   Accessible where wheeled stretchers might not be.

3. Stair chair

    i.   Excellent for staircases, small elevators, etc.

    ii.   Does not allow for manual cervical spine protection, CPR, or artificial ventilation.

4. Backboard

    i.   Lightweight, used primarily for moving patients or for spinal motion restriction (per local protocol).

    ii.   Allows for CPR, artificial ventilation, and a four-person lift.

5. Basket stretcher/Stokes basket

    i.   Used to carry patients across uneven terrain.

    ii.   Useful for remote locations not accessible by wheeled stretcher.

6. Scoop stretcher

    i.   Most scoop stretchers separate into two long pieces (left and right, not top to bottom).

    ii.   Allows for easy positioning with minimal patient movement, such as hip fracture. Can reduce patient discomfort during movement compared to other techniques.

7. Neonatal isolette

    i.   Designed to keep neonatal patients warm during transport.

    ii.   Requires specialized training to operate.

8. Patient packaging for air medical transport

    i.   Patient must be decontaminated if there is a hazardous material exposure before loading them on the aircraft.

    ii.   Notify air medical crew ASAP of any special circumstances, such as a large patient, cardiac arrest patient, traction splint applied, combative patient, unstable airway, etc.

    iii.   Secure all loose equipment, blankets, etc., before approaching a running aircraft.

    iv.   **Never** approach the aircraft without pilot or air medical crew authorization.

    v.   **Never** approach a rotor wing aircraft from the rear. **Never** back up.

H. Special considerations

1. Bariatric (obese) patients

    i.   Obese patients pose additional challenges and risks to providers during lifting and movement.

    ii. Know the weight limits for your equipment (stretcher, backboard, etc.).

    iii. Request additional assistance.

    iv. Some EMS systems have special bariatric ambulances with specialized equipment, automated lifting systems, and wider stretchers capable of a greater weight capacity.

2. Skeletal abnormalities

    i.   Patients with an unusual curvature of the spine (kyphosis or lordosis) may not be capable of lying supine without special padding.

    ii. Follow local protocol regarding spinal motion restriction.

3. Pregnant patients

    i.   Patients in the later stages of pregnancy should not be placed supine due to the risk of supine hypotensive syndrome.

    ii. Place the pregnant patient on their left side. If patient has potential cervical spine trauma, tilt backboard to the left about 20 degrees.

VII. MEDICAL RESTRAINT

A. Laws and protocols vary widely. However, in general, patients may be forcibly restrained if they pose a significant, immediate threat to you, your partner, or others.

1. Restraining a patient against their will is a last resort.

2. Use-of-force doctrine.

    i.   The EMT must act reasonably to prevent harm to a patient being forcibly restrained.

    ii. Use of force must be protective, *not* punitive.

3. Anticipate and plan. Request law enforcement assistance. Know your local protocols. Contact medical direction when possible.

B. When restraining a patient

1. Get additional help whenever possible (at least five people are recommended).

2. Only attempt to restrain patients you are capable of overpowering with the resources available.

3. Use the minimum amount of force necessary to protect yourself, the patient, and others.

4. Position the patient to prevent suffocation, aspiration, or circulatory compromise.

5. Use soft, padded restraints. Avoid handcuffs, flex-cuffs, etc.

6. Monitor the patient's level of consciousness, airway, and distal circulation (below point of restraints) continuously.

7. Thoroughly document the reason for restraining the patient, the method of restraint, the duration of restraint, and frequent reassessment of the patient while restrained.

8. **Never** restrain a patient in the prone position, hogtie a patient, or leave a restrained patient unsupervised.

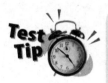

Security for the NREMT exam is rigorous. The questions on the exam come from an extensive unpublished database. Candidates cannot view the questions in advance. The only way to pass the test is to possess the necessary knowledge and exercise good test-taking skills. This *Crash Course* will help you with both!

PRACTICE QUESTIONS
Answers on page 380.

1. You are called to a business for a patient with dizziness, headache, and nausea. As you enter the business, you detect a strong odor and your eyes begin to water. You should immediately

A. leave the area and call for additional resources.

B. locate the patient and remove him.

C. apply a mask and goggles and treat the patient.

D. find the source of the odor and contain it.

2. Which of the following statements regarding stress is correct? (Select the THREE answer options that apply.)

   A. Stress is avoidable if you follow a few simple rules.

   B. Stress is unavoidable in the EMS profession.

   C. Acute stress develops slowly due to repeat exposure to certain events.

   D. EMTs can develop resiliency skills to manage stress.

   E. Exercise can help reduce stress.

   F. EMTs should avoid exercise while on duty.

3. Which of the following is a formalized process to help emergency responders deal with acute stress?

   A. paid time off

   B. modified duty assignment

   C. critical incident stress management

   D. EMS yoga

4. Which of the following provides the best protection from exposure to an airborne disease?

   A. handwashing

   B. face shield

   C. HEPA mask

   D. gloves

5. Which of the following moves is used when the scene is dangerous and the patient must be moved to safety before providing care?

   A. log roll

   B. emergency move

   C. rapid extrication

   D. power lift

Medical, Legal, and Ethical Issues, and EMS Research

I. TERMS TO KNOW

A. **Cultural competence:** Ability to provide care to patients with diverse values, beliefs, and behaviors.

B. **Health Insurance Portability and Accountability Act (HIPAA):** Federal law that requires the creation of national standards to protect sensitive patient health information from being disclosed.

C. **Negligence:** Deviation from the standard of care that a reasonable person would use in a particular set of circumstances.

D. **Scope of practice:** Outlines the actions a provider is legally allowed to perform based on certification/licensure.

E. **Standard of care:** Degree of care a reasonable person with similar training and experience would provide in a similar situation.

II. MEDICAL/LEGAL CONSIDERATIONS

A. Medical Direction and Medical Control

    1. Medical Direction: EMS providers operate under the direction of a physician medical director.

    2. Medical Control (online and offline)

        i. Direct or "online" medical control is provided over the phone or radio with a medical director or designated physician, such as at a base hospital.

        ii. Indirect or "offline" medical control is provided through written protocols.

3. Always contact your medical direction authority when you are unsure how to manage a patient.

B. Scope of Practice

1. Scope of practice outlines the actions a provider is legally allowed to perform based certification/licensure.

2. Scope of practice is tied to certification/licensure, not the individual's knowledge or experience.

3. Each state determines the scope of practice for its EMS providers.

C. Standard of Care

1. Standard of care is the degree of care a reasonable person with similar training and experience would provide in a similar situation.

2. Standard of care requires EMTs to competently perform the indicated assessment and treatment within their scope of practice.

3. All of the following can influence an EMT's standard of care:

   i. National EMS Education Standards

   ii. State protocols and guidelines

   iii. Medical direction

   iv. Employer's policies and procedures

   v. Reputable textbooks

   vi. Care considered acceptable by equivalent providers in the same community

Note: Think of scope of practice as what you are allowed to do. Think of standard of care as how well you need to be able to do it.

D. Consent

1. Informed consent

   i. Required from all patients who are alert and competent.

   ii. Patient must be informed of your care plan and associated risks of accepting or refusing care and transport.

   iii. Patient must be informed of, and understand, all information which would impact a reasonable person's decision to accept or refuse care and transport.

2. Express consent

    i.   Patient must be alert and competent.

    ii.   Can be given verbally or nonverbally.

    iii. Similar to informed consent, but not as in-depth.

    iv. Often used for more basic assessments or procedures.

3. Implied consent

    i.   Allows assumption of consent for emergency care of an unresponsive or incompetent patient.

    ii.   Incompetence may be due to alcohol, drugs, head injury, hypoxia, hypoglycemia, or mental incompetency.

    iii. Can be used for patients who initially refuse care, but later lose consciousness or become otherwise incapacitated.

4. Minor consent

    i.   Minors are not considered competent to give or refuse care.

    ii.   Consent required from parent or guardian.

        ➤ Implied consent can be used when unable to reach parent or guardian and treatment is needed.

        ➤ Minor consent is not required for emancipated minors. Criteria for emancipation varies, but usually includes minors who are married or pregnant, already a parent, a member of the armed forces, financially independent, or emancipated by the courts.

5. Involuntary consent

    i.   This is used for mentally incompetent adults or those in custody of law enforcement.

    ii.   Consent must be obtained from the entity with the appropriate legal authority.

E. Advance Directives

1. Written instructions, signed by the patient, specifying the patient's wishes regarding treatment and resuscitative efforts. There are different types of advance directives:

    i.   Do Not Resuscitate (DNR): DNR orders are specific to resuscitation efforts and do not affect treatment prior to the patient entering cardiac arrest.

ii. Living Will: Living wills are broader than DNRs and address healthcare wishes prior to entering cardiac arrest.

2. Requirements for legally recognized advance directive vary by state. Follow local protocol.

F. EMT Liability

1. Good Samaritan laws

   i. Good Samaritan laws are designed to protect those who render care without being compensated and or committing gross negligence.

   ii. Some states extend the Good Samaritan law to healthcare providers under certain conditions.

2. Criminal liability

   i. Criminal laws involve a government entity taking legal action against a person.

   ii. EMTs who are found criminally liable may face prison and/or loss of licensure.

   iii. Assault and battery

      ➤ Assault: A person can be guilty of assault even if another person only *perceives* an intent to inflict harm.

      ➤ Battery: The physical touching of another person without consent.

3. Civil liability

   i. In civil law, a plaintiff sues a defendant, such as an EMT, for a wrongful act involving injury or damage. The plaintiff seeks monetary compensation from the defendant.

   ii. A civil suit may involve multiple EMS providers, employers, the medical director, and others.

4. Negligence

   i. Negligence is the most common reason EMS providers are sued civilly.

      ➤ The EMS provider is accused of unintentional harm to the plaintiff.

      ➤ The plaintiff has the burden of proof, not the EMS provider.

ii.   The plaintiff must prove all four of the following:

➤ Duty to act: An obligation to respond and provide care.

➤ Breach of duty: Failure to assess, treat, or transport the patient according to the standard of care.

➤ Damage: Plaintiff experienced damage or injury worthy of compensation.

➤ Causation (also called *proximate cause*): The injury to the plaintiff was, at least in part, caused by the EMT's breach of duty.

5. Gross negligence

i.   Exceeds simple negligence. It involves an indifference to, and violation of, legal responsibility. Example: patient care that is reckless and presents a clear danger to the patient.

ii.   Can result in civil and/or criminal charges against the defendant.

6. Abandonment

i.   Abandonment is a form of negligence. It is the termination of care without transferring the patient to an equal or higher level of care.

ii.   Once care is initiated, EMS providers cannot unilaterally terminate care when continued care is still needed.

iii.   EMS example of abandonment: EMTs drop off a patient at the hospital without providing a transfer-of-care report.

iv.   *Note:* Paramedics **can** transfer care to EMTs if the paramedic has not initiated any advanced care that cannot be monitored or continued by the EMTs. Follow local protocol.

v.   Some protocols require online medical direction prior to terminating care.

vi.   Some state laws forbid EMS providers from discouraging patients to go by ambulance to the hospital.

7. False imprisonment/kidnapping

i.   EMS providers may be guilty of false imprisonment or kidnapping if they restrain or transport a competent patient against their will.

8. Hospital destination

    i.   Hospital destination and hospital diversion are common causes of lawsuits against EMS providers.

    ii.   Follow local protocols and national standards. When in doubt, consult medical direction.

    iii.   A patient's ability to pay should **not** figure into where a patient is transported.

    iv.   Clearly document why the destination facility was chosen, especially if you bypass a closer hospital.

9. Patient Refusals

    i.   Competent patients may refuse treatment regardless of the severity of their condition. Competency typically requires that the patient:

> Be alert to person, place, time, and events.

> Be of legal age.

> Understand what is happening and have no communication barriers, such as language or hearing.

> Not be impaired by drugs or alcohol.

> Not be mentally impaired due to significant illness or injury.

    ii.   Patients refusing treatment and transport must be fully informed of the treatment recommendations and the possible consequences of refusing treatment.

    iii.   Refusals present a high liability risk for EMS providers. Negligence or abandonment are much easier to prove if the patient is not transported.

    iv.   When confronted with a refusal, the EMT should:

> Do your best to talk the patient into treatment and transport.

> Follow your protocols.

> Consider requesting ALS backup.

> Contact medical direction for advice.

> Ensure the patient is making an informed refusal.

> Thoroughly document the incident using your agency's refusal form and obtain a signature from the patient and a witness if possible.

G. Patient Confidentiality

1. In most cases, EMS providers cannot release confidential information without the patient's consent.

    i. EMTs **can** release confidential information without consent when:

        ➤ The information is necessary for continuity of care.

        ➤ The information is necessary to facilitate billing for services.

        ➤ The EMT has received a subpoena.

        ➤ Reporting a possible crime, abuse, assault, negligence, certain injuries, or communicable diseases.

    ii. Health Insurance Portability and Accountability Act (HIPAA)

        ➤ Federal law established in 1996 which significantly changed healthcare practices in the U.S.

        ➤ Improved privacy protection of patient healthcare records.

        ➤ Gives patients greater control over how healthcare records are used and transferred.

        ➤ EMS employers are required to provide HIPAA training to all employees who have any contact with patients or patient records.

        ➤ EMS providers must provide patients with privacy practices and obtain signature of receipt.

H. COBRA and EMTALA

1. Consolidated Omnibus Budget Reconciliation Act (COBRA) and Emergency Medical Treatment and Active Labor Act (EMTALA)

    i. Both federal laws include regulations guaranteeing public access to emergency care.

    ii. Both laws are intended to stop the inappropriate transfer of patients.

2. COBRA and EMTALA are intended to prevent "patient dumping," which is considered a form of economic discrimination.

I. Interfacility Transports

1. The EMT must obtain a transfer report from the transferring facility before departing.

2. Confirm the exact location of the destination, including department or admitting physician.

3. Make sure the patient's needs don't exceed your scope of practice.

4. Obtain consent from the patient or guardian.

J. Death Determination

1. Local protocols vary on whether EMS providers have the authority to declare death. Follow local protocol. When in doubt, consult medical direction.

i. The following are typically considered obvious, definitive signs of death and thus resuscitation should *not* be initiated:

➤ Decapitation: The patient's head is no longer attached to the body.

➤ Decomposition: Physical decay of a dead body.

➤ Rigor mortis: Stiffening of the body after death.

➤ Dependent lividity: Settling of blood within the body.

K. Notification of Authorities. Law enforcement or the medical examiner's office must typically be notified about situations involving the following:

1. A deceased person

2. Suicide attempts

3. Assault, sexual assault

4. Child or elder abuse or neglect

5. Suspected crime scene

L. Organ Donors

1. Usually discovered through signed donor card or driver's license.

2. Treat the patient as you normally would and notify receiving personnel at the hospital.

M. Crime Scenes

1. Ensure scene safety.

2. After scene safety, the EMT's priority is patient care.

3. Avoid disturbing the crime scene any more than necessary to care for patients.

4. Remember to document the position of patient(s) and everything you touched.

5. Cut around (not through) holes in clothing when exposing the patient.

6. Report anyone or anything that seems suspicious to law enforcement.

7. Discourage sexual assault patients from changing clothes, showering, etc., until law enforcement arrives.

8. Try to have same-sex provider assist with sexual assault victims.

9. Leave once you are no longer needed at the scene.

III. PROFESSIONAL ETHICS IN EMS

A. Ethics are the moral principles that guide a person or group, such as the healthcare profession (known as bioethics).

B. Every EMS call presents some sort of ethical issue or consideration.

C. An EMT's professional ethics should reflect what is described in the EMT Code of Ethics published by the National Association of EMTs.

D. Personal morals, professional ethics, and the law

1. An EMT's moral, ethical, and legal obligations do not usually conflict with one another. For example, all three should require that you document factually the care you provided, not the care you should have provided.

2. When conflicts arise . . .

   i. Consider what is best for the patient.

   ii. Know the law and your protocols.

   iii. Get help (partner, supervisor, ALS personnel, medical direction, etc.).

E. Cultural Competency

1. Cultural competence in healthcare describes the ability to provide care to patients with diverse values, beliefs, and behaviors.

2. Cultural competence improves both patient care and patient safety.

3. At-risk patients and those with healthcare disparities:

    i. Economically disadvantaged

    ii. Minorities

    iii. Victims of domestic violence and human trafficking

    iv. Pediatrics and geriatrics

    v. Patients with special healthcare needs

    vi. Patients who need chronic or end-of-life care

IV. EMS RESEARCH

A. Historical EMS protocols

1. In the past, EMS protocols were based almost entirely on recommendations from physicians.

2. Often, these recommendations were based on in-hospital practices rather than the prehospital environment.

3. In some cases, these practices did not improve outcomes in the prehospital environment, or even did harm.

B. Modern EMS protocols

1. Today, EMS treatment decisions come from evidence-based medicine.

2. The body of valid EMS-specific research is growing.

3. For more information on EMS research, visit the UCLA Prehospital Care Research Forum at *https://www.cpc.mednet.ucla.edu/pcrf.*

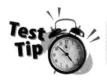

Test Tip

Multiple-response items (where you must select more than one answer) will always tell you how many answer options you need to select.

PRACTICE QUESTIONS
Answers on page 380.

1. Which of the following terms refers to the actions an EMT is legally allowed to perform based on their license or certification?

   A. duty to act

   B. standard of care

   C. scope of practice

   D. doctrine of certification

2. Which of the following terms refers to the degree of care a reasonable person with similar training should provide in a similar situation?

   A. standard of care

   B. scope of practice

   C. standardized care doctrine

   D. EMS expectation clause

3. Which of the following are specific to resuscitation efforts and do not affect treatment prior to the patient entering cardiac arrest?

   A. living will

   B. advance directive

   C. DNR order

   D. medical power of attorney

4. Which of the following must a plaintiff show when an EMT is accused of negligence? (Select the TWO answer options that apply.)

   A. The EMT showed willful disregard for the patient's well-being.

   B. The plaintiff's injury was due to the EMT's action or inaction.

   C. The damage to the plaintiff is worthy of financial compensation.

   D. The EMT was off duty when the incident occurred.

   E. The EMT did not contact medical direction for advice.

5. Which of the following is a definitive sign of death?

    A. decapitation

    B. pulselessness

    C. apnea

    D. unresponsiveness

Communications and Documentation

I. TERMS TO KNOW

A. **Empathy:** Ability to see things from the patient's perspective.

B. **E-PCR:** Electronic patient care report.

C. **Federal Communications Commission (FCC):** Federal agency that regulates all radio operations in the U.S.

D. **Telemedicine:** Delivery of healthcare services via telecommunication technologies.

E. **Therapeutic communication:** Techniques that prioritize the physical, mental, and emotional well-being of patients.

II. COMMUNICATIONS

A. Introduction to Communications

　1. EMS communications typically relate to mobile-based communications with dispatch, other emergency responders, medical direction, etc.

　2. Therapeutic communications typically relate to your interaction with the patient and ability to obtain clinical information.

　3. Interpersonal communication is the ability to send and receive information between at least two people.

B. EMS Communications

　1. Portable radios: Hand-held radios with a very limited range unless used with a repeater system.

2. Mobile radios: Vehicle-mounted radios with a greater range than portable radios; however, a repeater system is typically still required.

3. Base station: A transmitter/receiver; a fixed location that is in contact with all other components of the radio system.

4. Repeater: A type of base station that receives low-power transmissions from portable or mobile radios and rebroadcasts at higher power to significantly improve range.

5. Mobile data computers (MDCs)

   i. Relay digital information instead of voice transmissions. Reduces radio traffic.

   ii. Can display information such as address of call, routing information, call details, etc.

6. Cellphones

   i. Cellphones have largely replaced radios for communication with medical direction.

   ii. Advantages: Easy, clear audio quality, inexpensive.

   iii. Disadvantages: Potentially unreliable during peak demand or mass casualty incidents.

7. Federal Communications Commission (FCC)

   i. The FCC regulates all radio operations in the U.S.

   ii. FCC has allocated specific frequencies exclusively for EMS use.

C. Guidelines for Radio Communications

1. Communication with dispatch (typically done via MDC)

   i. Confirm receipt of dispatch information.

   ii. Notify dispatch when en route to call, on scene, en route to hospital, and at the hospital.

2. **Do . . .**

   i. make sure you are on the correct radio/frequency.

   ii. ensure there is no other radio traffic before transmitting.

   iii. depress push-to-talk (PTT) button for one second before speaking.

      iv. identify who you are talking to first, then say who you are. Example: "Dispatch, this is Medic 1."

      v. use clear text, not radio codes unless approved locally.

      vi. use "affirmative" and "negative" instead of "yes" and "no."

      vii. use "copy" to confirm receipt of a transmission.

      viii. always repeat ("echo") orders from medical direction to ensure accuracy.

3. **Do NOT . . .**

      i. use unnecessary verbiage, such as "please" or "thank you."

      ii. relay protected information such as the patient's name.

D. Communicating with Medical Direction

1. Communicating with medical direction typically involves relaying a large volume of information clearly in a short period of time.

2. Details matter and mutual understanding is critical.

3. Strong verbal communication skills are essential.

4. Provide objective (factual) information rather than subjective (opinions) information.

5. Each patient situation is unique; however, patient information should always be relayed in an organized manner, with the most important information first.

6. Sample format for relaying patient information

      i. Unit designation, certification level, destination, and estimated time of arrival

      ii. Patient's age, sex, chief complaint

      iii. Patient's level of consciousness (LOC), Glasgow Coma Scale (GCS) score, history of present illness (HPI) or mechanism of injury (MOI)

      iv. Any associated symptoms and pertinent negatives

      v. Vitals, physical examination

      vi. Patient's history, medications, allergies

      vii. Treatment initiated and response to treatment

      viii. Any requests for additional interventions

      ix. Echo any orders provided by medical direction

> **Note:** You may be guilty of abandonment if you do not provide a verbal transfer of care report to an equal or higher medical authority.

E. Transfer of Care

   1. Verbal report: Transfer of care must include a verbal report to an equal or higher medical authority. Provide all relevant information (similar to radio report), including any changes since radio report.

   2. A written copy of the patient care report must be provided.

   3. Obtain signature from accepting hospital provider verifying transfer of care.

F. Interpersonal Communication

   1. Sending and receiving verbal communication

      i. The message sender "encodes" the message, and the receiver "decodes" the message.

      ii. Senders and receivers trade roles frequently.

      iii. Radio communications can be limiting if only one person can send/receive at a time.

      iv. Often, what the sender intended to convey (imply) is not what the receiver interpreted (inferred).

   2. Factors that influence communication

      i. Nonverbal cues, such as body language. This is lost with radio/phone communication.

      ii. Perception of attitude and tone significantly impact effectiveness of communication.

   3. Establishing a rapport with the patient

      i. Introduce yourself, then ask for the patient's name and use it.

      ii. Make eye contact and be honest.

      iii. Use age-appropriate language and techniques.

      iv. Be aware of special needs, such as hearing impaired.

      v. Respect cultural differences.

vi. **Do NOT . . .**

> ➤ make false promises, lie, or mislead the patient.

> ➤ give advice or opinions beyond your scope of practice.

> ➤ use biased or judgmental language or questions.

> ➤ be confrontational or overexert your authority.

> ➤ overuse medical terms or lingo.

4. Challenging communications situations include:

   i. Patients with special challenges

   ii. Patients under the influence of drugs or alcohol

   iii. Pediatric patients

G. Therapeutic Communication

1. Compassion: Clearly convey your concern for the patient's well-being.

2. Empathy: Work to see things from the patient's perspective.

3. Competence: Communicate competence through your words and actions.

4. Confidence: Communicate that you are a professional and you know what needs to be done.

5. Conscience: Communicate that you are adhering to the ethical standards of your profession.

6. Commitment: Communicate that you are committed to whatever is best for the patient.

7. When questioning patients . . .

   i. Listen!

   ii. Ask the important questions first.

   iii. Use open-ended questions when possible. Example: "Can you tell us why you called today?" instead of, "Are you having chest pain?"

   iv. Use closed questions (yes or no) when you need specific information quickly.

   v. Avoid judgmental or biased questions.

H. Emerging communications technologies

1. Telemedicine: Provides real-time, two-way audio and video communication between those on scene and physicians, such as medical control at a base hospital. This is a great tool for high-risk patient refusals.

2. Mobile integrated healthcare: MIH is provided by a wide array of healthcare entities and practitioners that are administratively or clinically integrated with EMS agencies.

III. DOCUMENTATION

A. Purposes of the Patient Care Report

1. Continuity of care: Provides information to those that will continue care of patient.

2. Legal document

   i. PCR becomes part of the patient's permanent medical record.

   ii. Typically, the person who wrote the PCR will be the person subpoenaed to give a deposition or testify in court.

   iii. **Documentation Rule No. 1:** If you did it, document it. If you didn't do it, don't say that you did.

   iv. **Documentation Rule No. 2:** It is much better to document well than to explain later why you didn't do so.

3. Billing: The PCR may be used to bill the patient or insurance provider.

4. Research and quality improvement.

B. Minimum data set: Information that should be included on every PCR

1. Times: Dispatch time, time en route to call, time on scene, patient contact time, time en route to hospital, arrival time at hospital, time transfer of care was completed.

   i. Accurate times are critical. Synchronize clocks on medical devices, watches, phones, etc., with dispatch center.

   ii. Inaccurate times are an easy target for litigators.

   iii. **Documentation Rule No. 3:** If your times are inaccurate, the rest of your PCR may be called into question.

2. Patient information: Age, sex, chief complaint, level of consciousness, vitals (at least two sets), all assessments, treatment, and response to treatment.

3. Administrative info: Address and date of call, unit designation, name and identifying number and certification level of all EMS providers on the call.

4. Narrative: This is where the EMT can "paint the picture" of what happened during the call.

C. Documentation Guidelines and Formats

1. FACT documentation

   i. Factual: The PCR should be fact-based, not opinion-based.

   ii. Accurate: The PCR should be as accurate as possible. Never falsify a PCR.

   iii. Complete: The PCR should be as complete as possible. If something wasn't completed, document why.

   iv. Timely: The PCR should be completed as soon as possible after the transfer of care. It is a good idea to document when the PCR was completed.

2. SOAP documentation format

   i. Subjective

     ➤ Chief complaint

     ➤ HPI

     ➤ History

     ➤ Medications

     ➤ Allergies

   ii. Objective

     ➤ Vitals

     ➤ Physical exam

     ➤ Other diagnostic data

   iii. Assessment

     ➤ Combines subjective and objective data

     ➤ Document possible problems, field impression

    iv. Plan

       ➤ Treatment initiated

       ➤ Response to treatment

3. CHART documentation format

    i.   Chief complaint

    ii. History

    iii. Assessment: head, eyes, ears, nose, throat (HEENT) exam; chest/back; abdomen; extremities

    iv. **Rx:** treatments and response to treatments

    v.   Transport: changes during transport

4. Associated symptoms and pertinent negatives

    i.   Associated symptoms: Patient complaints that are in addition to the chief complaint. For example, the chief complaint is chest pain, but the patient also complains of mild difficulty breathing.

    ii. Pertinent negatives: Signs or symptoms you have reason to suspect, but the patient denies. Example: The patient experienced trauma but denies neck pain, or the patient has chest pain but denies dyspnea.

5. Abbreviations and spelling

    i.   Most agencies have a list of approved abbreviations. Avoid using abbreviations not on your employer's list.

    ii. **Documentation Rule No. 4:** Spelling counts!

6. Errors and falsifications

    i.   Most PCRs are now completed electronically; however, if you discover a handwritten mistake, draw a single line through it and make the correction. Never scribble out a mistake so it cannot be read.

    ii. Intentional falsification of a PCR is a serious ethical violation. It compromises patient care. It is grounds for termination, revocation of certification/licensure, and possible legal action.

    iii. Errors of omission and commission

       ➤ Errors of omission: Something that should have been included on the PCR was left out.

➤ Errors of commission: Something was included on the PCR that is incorrect.

5. Patient refusals

    i.   Thoroughly document the patient's competency.

    ii.   Thoroughly document your assessments, treatments, and response to treatments. If something that should have been completed was not, document why. Example: "Patient refused vitals assessment."

    iii.   Document any assessments or treatments that the patient refused.

    iv.   Document at least two sets of vitals, or document why you did not.

    v.   Document your recommendations regarding treatment and transport.

    vi.   Document your discussion about the risks of refusing treatment and transport.

    vii.   Document that the patient understood all of the information provided and made an informed decision to refuse treatment and transport.

    viii.   Document your discussion with medical direction.

    ix.   Document your recommendation that the patient can call again at any time.

    x.   Obtain a signature from the patient on the refusal form, or document why it was not obtained.

    xi.   Obtain a signature from a witness, but not a fellow EMS provider.

D. Possible Special Reporting Situations

1. Death

2. Mass casualty incidents

3. Suspected abuse or neglect

4. Suspected crime

5. Animal bites

6. Disease outbreak

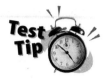

PRACTICE QUESTIONS
Answers on page 381.

1. What federal agency regulates all radio communications in the United States?

    A. Federal Trade Commission (FTC)

    B. Department of Transportation (DOT)

    C. National Registry of EMTs (NREMT)

    D. Federal Communications Commission (FCC)

2. Which of the following statements is correct regarding EMS radio communications?

    A. Begin and end radio transmissions with "please" and "thank you."

    B. Use the 10-codes approved by the NREMT.

    C. Use clear text, not radio codes.

    D. State "over and out" at the end of each transmission.

3. Which of the following are examples of objective observation? (Select the TWO answer options that apply.)

    A. "The patient has slurred speech."

    B. "The patient is high on something."

    C. "The patient is obviously intoxicated."

    D. "The patient is under the influence of drugs."

    E. "The patient is unresponsive to pain."

4. Which of the following suggestions is appropriate?

    A. If you didn't do it, don't document that you did.

    B. Always keep a copy of your PCR for your own records.

    C. Have your patient review the PCR once it is complete.

    D. Leave your name off the PCR if you have concerns about the call.

5. What abbreviations should you use on the PCR?

    A. You can use any abbreviations that are legible.

    B. Abbreviations are never allowed on the PCR.

    C. Only use abbreviations approved by the NREMT.

    D. Use only abbreviations approved by your agency.

Anatomy and Physiology/ Medical Terminology

 I. **TERMS TO KNOW**

    A. **Anatomy:** Study of the structure of the body.

    B. **Homeostasis:** Self-regulating process where the body functions optimally while adjusting to varying conditions.

    C. **Pathophysiology:** Study of disease or injury.

    D. **Perfusion:** Adequate circulation of blood throughout the body.

    E. **Physiology:** Study of the function of the body.

    F. **Shock:** Inadequate perfusion.

II. **KEY TOPICS**

    A. Anatomy: the study of the body's structure

    B. Physiology: the study of the body's function

    C. Pathophysiology: the study of disease

 III. **HOMEOSTASIS**

    A. Homeostasis is a state of balance or equilibrium within the body.

    B. Every cell, tissue, organ, and system in the human body functions to maintain homeostasis.

    C. The human body's homeostatic range is quite narrow.

IV. TOPOGRAPHIC ANATOMY

A. There are numerous terms used to reference locations on the outer surface of the body. All terms are based on the body being in the "anatomical position."

B. Anatomical position: The body is in the standing position, arms at the sides, with palms forward (thumbs on the outside).

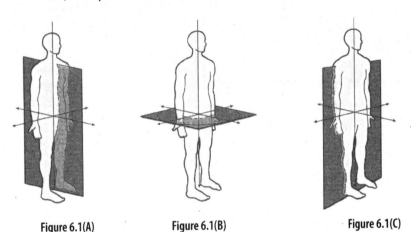

| Figure 6.1(A) | Figure 6.1(B) | Figure 6.1(C) |

C. Planes of the Body

1. The midline divides the body into left and right. (A)

2. The transverse plane divides the body into top and bottom at the level of the umbilicus (belly button). (B)

3. The frontal plane (imaginary line) divides the body into anterior and posterior. (C)

D. Paired Directional Terms

1. Anterior or ventral (front) and posterior or dorsal (back)

2. Superior (top) and inferior (bottom)

3. Proximal (closer to point of attachment) and distal (farther from point of attachment)

4. Medial (close to midline) and lateral (far from midline)

E. Terms of Movement

1. Abduction: movement away from midline

    i. Example: Assume the anatomical position; lift your arms straight up at your sides (not in front of you). This is abduction.

2. Adduction: movement toward the midline

    i. Example: With your arms straight out at your sides, move them down to anatomical position. This is adduction.

3. Extension: straightening the joint (increasing the angle of the joint).

    i. Example: Bend your arm so there is a 90-degree angle between your forearm and upper arm (flexed bicep position). Extend the arm so both portions of the arm form a straight line. This is extension.

4. Flexion: bending the joint (decreasing the angle of the joint).

    i. Example: Stand in the anatomical position. Leave your upper leg in position, bend at the knee, and lift the lower leg up behind you. This is flexion.

F. Body Positions

1. Supine: lying on you back, face up

2. Prone: lying on your stomach, face down

3. Fowler position: seated with head elevated

4. Recovery position: lying on the left or right side

Note: The use of Trendelenburg or "shock position" is no longer recommended.

G. Abdominal Quadrants. The four abdominal quadrants are based on the intersection of the midline and the transverse line. Remember that *left* and *right* are **always** in reference to the patient's left and right.

1. Left upper quadrant (LUQ)

2. Right upper quadrant (RUQ)

3. Left lower quadrant (LLQ)

4. Right lower quadrant (RLQ)

V. SKELETAL SYSTEM

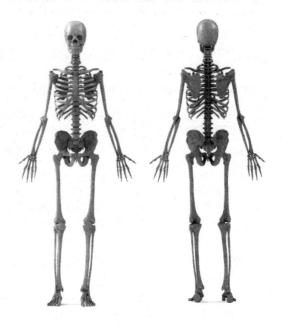

Figure 6.2

A. The skeletal system provides shape, allows movement, and protects internal organs.

B. There are 206 bones in the human body.

C. Tendons, ligaments, and cartilage are also part of the skeletal system.

   1. Ligaments connect bone to bone.

   2. Tendons connect bone muscle.

   3. Cartilage is connective tissue that allows smooth movement of joints.

D. Axial Skeleton. The axial skeleton consists primarily of the skull, spinal column, and ribcage (thoracic cavity).

   1. Skull

      i.   Frontal bone: the forehead

      ii. Parietal bone: top of head, between frontal and occipital bones

  iii. Occipital bone: posterior portion of the skull

  iv. Temporal bone: lateral bones, above the cheekbones

  v. Maxillae: forms the upper jaw, above upper teeth

  vi. Mandible: movable portion of lower jaw

  vii. Zygomatic bone: cheekbones

  viii. Nasal bone: the nose

  ix. Foramen magnum: opening in the occipital bone where brain connects to spinal cord

 2. Spinal column

  i. Central supporting structure; protects the spinal cord

  ii. Consists of 33 vertebrae (9 of them are fused)

  iii. The spinal column in descending order (superior to inferior):

   ➤ Cervical spine: 7 vertebrae, C1 to C7

   ➤ Thoracic spine: 12 vertebrae, T1 to T12

   ➤ Lumbar spine: 5 vertebrae, L1 to L5

   ➤ Sacrum: 5 fused vertebrae

   ➤ Coccyx: 4 fused vertebrae

 3. Thoracic cavity

  i. Houses the heart, lungs, trachea, esophagus, and great vessels

  ii. Sternum: breastbone

   ➤ Manubrium: upper portion of the sternum

   ➤ Body: middle portion of the sternum

   ➤ Xiphoid process: inferior tip of the sternum

E. Appendicular Skeleton

 1. Includes the bones of the arms, legs, and pelvis

 2. Shoulder girdle: formed by the clavicle (collarbone), scapula (shoulder blade), humerus (upper arm)

 3. Arm

  i. Humerus: upper arm

  ii. Radius: lateral bone of forearm (thumb side)

      iii. Ulna: medial bone of forearm

      iv. Carpal bones (wrist)

      v. Metacarpals (base of the fingers)

      vi. Phalanges (fingers)

  4. Pelvis: a ring-shaped structure formed by three bones

      i. Illium: upper portion of the pelvis

      ii. Ischium: lower portion of the pelvis

      iii. Pubis: anterior portion of the pelvis

  5. Leg

      i. Femur: thigh bone (the strongest bone of the body)

      ii. Patella: kneecap

      iii. Tibia: medial bone of the lower leg (shinbone)

      iv. Fibula: lateral bone of the lower leg

      v. Tarsal bones (ankle)

      vi. Metatarsal (base of the toes)

      vii. Phalanges (toes)

  6. Joints. A joint exists where two long bones come together.

      i. Symphysis: a joint with limited motion

      ii. Ball-and-socket joint: a joint where the distal end is capable of free motion, such as the shoulder

      iii. Hinge joint: a joint where the bones can move only uniaxially, such as the knee

F. Muscles. There are three types of muscles.

  1. Smooth muscle: involuntary muscle located within the blood vessels and the digestive tract

  2. Skeletal: voluntary muscle that attaches to the skeleton

      i. Biceps: anterior humerus

      ii. Triceps: posterior humerus

      iii. Pectoralis: anterior chest

    iv. Latissimus dorsi: posterior chest

    v. Rectus abdominis: abdominal muscles

    vi. Quadriceps (four muscles): anterior femur

    vii. Biceps femoris: posterior femur; part of hamstring muscle

    viii. Gluteus (three muscles): buttocks

  3. Cardiac: heart muscle

VI. RESPIRATORY SYSTEM

A. The respiratory system provides the body with adequate oxygen and eliminates waste products such as carbon dioxide (CO_2). The respiratory system helps regulate pH levels to assist in maintaining homeostasis.

B. Upper Airway

  1. Components of the upper airway include:

    i. nose and mouth

    ii. nasopharynx (upper part of the throat behind the nose)

    iii. oropharynx (area of the throat behind the mouth)

    iv. larynx (voice box)

    v. epiglottis (valve that protects the opening of the trachea)

  2. Most of the manual airway techniques and mechanical airway adjuncts used by the EMT are designed to clear and protect the upper airway.

  3. Foreign-body airway obstruction (FBAO) is a concern for the EMT. The tongue is by far the most common cause of upper-airway obstruction.

C. Lower Airway

  1. Components of lower airway include:

    i. trachea

    ii. carina (where the trachea branches into left and right mainstem bronchi)

    iii. left and right mainstem bronchi (primary branches of the trachea leading to left and right lungs)

    iv. bronchioles (smaller branches of the bronchi)

    v. alveoli

> ➤ All airway structures above the alveoli serve to get air to this point in the respiratory system.

> ➤ This is the only place in the respiratory system where oxygen and carbon dioxide are exchanged.

> ➤ Alveoli are in contact with pulmonary capillaries.

> ➤ Pulmonary capillaries diffuse carbon dioxide from the body to the alveoli.

> ➤ Alveoli diffuse oxygen from the respiratory system to the body.

> ➤ Surfactant is a substance that helps keep the alveoli from collapsing.

D. Lung Expansion

1. Pleura: two thin, smooth layers of tissue with thin film of fluid in between to allow frictionless movement across one another

    i. Visceral pleura: lines the outer surface of the lungs

    ii. Parietal pleura: lines the inside surface of the chest cavity

2. During inhalation, as the chest expands, the parietal pleura pull the visceral pleura, which pull the lungs.

E. Muscles of Breathing

1. Diaphragm

    i. The diaphragm is the primary muscle of respiration.

    ii. It separates the thoracic cavity from the abdominal cavity.

    iii. It is usually under involuntary control but can be controlled voluntarily.

    iv. The esophagus and great vessels pass through the diaphragm.

    v. The diaphragm is dome shaped until it contracts during inhalation. During inhalation, it moves down and expands the size of the thoracic cavity.

2. Intercostal muscles. Located between the ribs, the intercostal muscles contract during inhalation and expand the thoracic cage.

3. Respiration and ventilation

   i. In general, the terms "respiration," "ventilation," and "breathing" refer to the movement of air in and out of the lungs. Although they are often used synonymously, there are some distinctions to be made. Ventilation is also called pulmonary ventilation.

   ii. Inhalation through negative pressure breathing

   ➤ The diaphragm and intercostal muscles contract, the thoracic cage expands, pressure in the chest cavity decreases, and air rushes in.

   ➤ Inhalation is an active process and requires energy.

   ➤ Atmospheric air contains 21% oxygen.

   iii. Exhalation

   ➤ The diaphragm and intercostal muscles relax, the thoracic cage contracts, pressure in the chest cavity rises, and air is expelled.

   ➤ Exhalation is normally passive and does not require energy.

   ➤ Exhaled air contains 16% oxygen.

   iv. External respiration: the exchange of oxygen and carbon dioxide between the alveoli and pulmonary capillaries

   v. Internal respiration: gas exchanged between the body's cells and the systemic capillaries

   vi. Cellular respiration (better known as aerobic metabolism): uses oxygen to break down glucose to create energy

F. Carbon Dioxide Drive

   1. This is the primary mechanism of breathing control for most people.

   2. The brain stem monitors carbon dioxide (CO_2) levels in the blood and cerebrospinal fluid.

   3. High CO_2 levels will stimulate an increase in respiratory rate and tidal volume.

G. Hypoxic Drive

    1. Hypoxic drive is a backup system to the CO_2 drive.

    2. Specialized sensors in the brain, aorta, and carotid arteries monitor oxygen levels.

    3. Low oxygen levels will stimulate breathing.

    4. The hypoxic drive is less effective than CO_2 drive.

H. Lung Volumes

    1. Tidal volume: the amount of air inhaled or exhaled in one breath.

    2. Residual volume: the amount of air in the lungs after completely exhaling. The residual volume keeps the lungs open.

    3. Inspiratory and expiratory reserve volume: the amount of air you can still inhale or exhale after a normal breath.

    4. Dead space: the amount of air in the respiratory system not including the alveoli.

    5. Minute volume: respiratory rate × tidal volume.

I. Normal Breathing

    1. Normal rate and tidal volume

        i. Normal adult rate: 12 to 20 breaths per minute (bpm)

        ii. Normal pediatric rate: 15 to 30 bpm

        iii. Normal infant rate: 25 to 50 bpm

    2. Non-labored

    3. Regular rhythm

    4. Clear and equal breath sounds bilaterally

J. Abnormal Breathing

    1. Abnormal rate or tidal volume

    2. Labored breathing

    3. Muscle retractions

        i. Intercostal retractions: between the ribs

        ii. Supraclavicular retractions: above the clavicles

        iii. Use of abdominal muscles

4. Abnormal skin color

5. Tripod position: seated, leaning forward, and using the arms to help breath

6. Agonal breaths: dying gasps; slow and shallow; will not move air into alveoli

VII. CIRCULATORY SYSTEM

A. The circulatory system includes all blood vessels, capillaries, and the heart. It is also called the cardiovascular system.

B. The Heart

1. A muscular organ with two pumps, one on the left side and another on the right

   i. The left pump receives oxygenated blood from the lungs and sends it throughout the body. It is the stronger of the two pumps, with a greater workload than the right pump.

   ii. The right pump receives deoxygenated blood from the body and sends it to the lungs to drop off carbon dioxide and pick up oxygen on its way to the left heart.

   iii. A septal wall divides the heart into left and right sides.

2. The heart walls contain three layers enclosed in the pericardium, a fibrous sac that surrounds the heart. From inner to outer, the layers are:

   i. Endocardium: the smooth, thin lining on the inside of the heart

   ii. Myocardium: the thick middle, muscular layer of the heart

   iii. Epicardium: the outermost layer of the heart and innermost layer of the pericardium

3. The chambers and valves

   i. Atria: the two upper chambers of the heart. Blood returning to the heart on both sides enters the atria (atrium). The atria pump the blood into the ventricles just before the ventricles contract. This is called the "atrial kick" and helps increase cardiac output.

   ii. Ventricles: the lower and larger chambers of the heart. Ventricles receive blood from the atria and send it out of the heart during ventricular contraction. Under normal circumstances, this generates a palpable pulse. The left ventricle sends oxygen-rich blood throughout the body under high pressure. The right ventricle sends oxygen-depleted blood to the lungs under low pressure.

iii. Heart valves: one-way valves between the atria and ventricles that allow blood to move in a downward direction into the ventricles during atrial contraction. The valves then close during ventricular contraction to prevent regurgitation of blood back into the atria.

4. Cardiac conduction system

i. The heart has its own electrical system. It generates electrical impulses, which stimulate contraction of the heart muscle.

ii. The heart can generate electrical impulses from three different locations. The primary power plant, the sinoatrial (SA) node, normally generates impulses between 60 to 100 times per minute in the adult. That's why the normal heart rate in adults is 60 to 100 beats per minute.

➤ The atrioventricular (AV) junction is the backup pacemaker and generates electrical impulses at about 40 to 60 per minute.

➤ The bundle of His is the final pacemaker for the heart. It generates impulses only at about 20 to 40 per minute.

iii. The heart, like the brain, is extremely intolerant of a lack of oxygen. The heart receives its blood flow from the coronary arteries, which branch off from the aorta.

iv. Cardiac output (circulation) will cease if the heart is unable to generate electrical impulses or if the heart muscle is too damaged to respond to the impulses.

5. Cardiac contraction

i. Myocardial contractility

➤ Contractility refers to the heart's ability to contract.

➤ Adequate contractility requires adequate blood volume and muscle strength.

ii. Preload

➤ Preload is the precontraction pressure based on the amount of blood coming back to the heart.

➤ Increased preload leads to increased stretching of the ventricles and increased myocardial contractility.

iii. Afterload

➤ Afterload is the resistance the heart must overcome during ventricular contraction.

➤ Increased afterload leads to decreased cardiac output.

The Pathway of Blood Flow Through the Heart

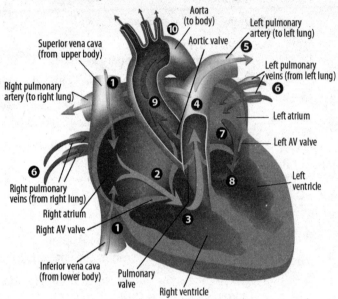

Figure 6.3

C. Blood Flow Through the Cardiovascular System

1. Oxygen-rich blood exits the left heart through the aorta. The aorta branches off into arteries, then arterioles, and finally capillaries. On the venous side, capillaries feed into venules, then veins, and finally the superior or inferior vena cava.

2. In Figure 6.3, the vena cava (1) returns blood to the right side of the heart into the right atrium (2). The right atrium pumps blood into the right ventricle (3), which pumps deoxygenated blood through the pulmonary arteries (4 and 5) into the lungs. The carbon dioxide and oxygen exchange takes place between the alveoli and the pulmonary capillaries. Oxygen-rich blood from the lungs returns to the left heart through the pulmonary veins (6) into the left atrium (7). The left atrium pumps blood into the

left ventricle (8), which then pumps it to the aorta (9 and 10) for circulation throughout the body.

3. Arteries always carry blood away from the heart, and veins always carry blood toward the heart. *Note:* The pulmonary artery is the one artery in the body that carries deoxygenated blood. The pulmonary vein is the only vein in the body that carries oxygen-rich blood.

4. Systemic vascular resistance (SVR)

    i.   SVR is the resistance to blood flow throughout the body (excluding the pulmonary system).

    ii. SVR is determined by the size of blood vessels:

       ➤ Constriction (reduced size) of blood vessels increases SVR and can cause an increase in blood pressure.

       ➤ Dilation (increased size) of blood vessels decreases SVR and can lower blood pressure.

D. Arterial Pulses

  1. Central pulses

    i.   Carotid pulse: can be felt by palpating the carotid artery in the neck during contraction of the left ventricle

    ii. Femoral: can be felt by palpating the femoral artery in the groin area during contraction of the left ventricle

  2. Peripheral pulses

    i.   Radial pulse: palpated in the wrist on the radial (thumb) side

    ii. Brachial pulse: palpated on the medial portion of the upper arm beneath the biceps muscle; can also be felt on the anterior medial area of the arm where the humerus meets the forearm (elbow area)

    iii. Dorsalis pedis: palpated on top of the foot

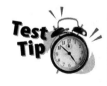

Test Tip

It takes a lot to memorize how blood flows through the circulatory system, including the heart's chambers and valves, but it is worth the effort! With this knowledge, you are likely to answer a few more questions correctly on the NREMT exam. You will also be better able to distinguish the signs of left-sided heart failure from right-sided heart failure in the field.

VIII. BLOOD, BLOOD PRESSURE, AND PERFUSION

A. Components of Blood

1. Plasma: the liquid component of blood; made mostly of water

2. Red blood cells (erythrocytes): the oxygen-carrying component of blood

3. White blood cells (leukocytes): fight infection by defending against invading organisms

4. Platelets: essential for clot formation to stop bleeding

B. Blood Pressure. Blood pressure is a measurement of the pressure exerted against the walls of the arteries.

1. Systolic pressure: the blood pressure exerted during contraction of the left ventricle

2. Diastolic pressure: the blood pressure in between contractions

C. Perfusion. Perfusion is the flow of blood throughout the body.

1. Adequate perfusion means blood flow is adequate to all the tissues and organs in the body.

2. Inadequate perfusion (hypoperfusion or shock) means blood flow has been compromised to the point the entire body is at risk.

IX. NERVOUS SYSTEM

A. Structural and Functional Divisions of the Nervous System

1. Central nervous system (CNS)

    i. The CNS consists of the brain and spinal cord.

    ii. The CNS is the command and control portion of the nervous system.

    iii. The brain receives information from the peripheral nervous system (PNS), makes decisions, and sends orders to the PNS.

    iv. Parts of the brain

        ➤ Cerebrum: largest part of the brain; controls thought, memory, and the senses

> ➤ Cerebellum: coordinates voluntary movement, fine motor function, and balance

> ➤ Brain stem: includes midbrain, pons, and medulla; controls essential body functions, such as breathing and consciousness

v. The spinal cord is the communication bridge between the brain and the PNS.

> ➤ Cerebrospinal fluid (CSF): a clear fluid in and around brain and spinal cord; cushions the CNS and filters contaminants

2. Peripheral nervous system

i. The PNS includes all other nervous system structures outside of the CNS, including cranial and peripheral nerves.

ii. The PNS sends information to the CNS and carries out orders from the CNS.

iii. Two divisions of the PNS

> ➤ Sensory division: sends sensory information to the CNS.

> ➤ Motor division: receives motor commands from the CNS. There are two divisions of the motor portion of PNS.

> — Somatic: voluntary portion of the PNS

> — Autonomic nervous system (ANS): involuntary portion of the PNS

>> a. Sympathetic: "fight-or-flight" portion of autonomic nervous system; exerts greater control in times of stress or danger

>> b. Parasympathetic: "feed-and-breed" portion of nervous system; exerts greater control in times of rest, digestion, or reproduction

X. INTEGUMENTARY SYSTEM (SKIN)

A. Epidermis

1. Outermost layer of the skin

2. Two epidermal layers

      i.   The germinal layer produces new cells and pushes them to the surface. The cells die en route to the surface.

      ii.   The stratum corneal layer is the top epidermal layer and consists of dead skin cells.

   3. Dermis. The dermis contains blood vessels, nerve endings, sweat glands, and hair follicles.

B. Subcutaneous Tissue

   1. Fatty tissue

   2. The deepest layer of the integumentary system, above the muscle layer

XI. ABDOMINAL CAVITY

A. The abdominal cavity contains numerous organs of digestion and excretion.

B. It is separated from the thoracic cavity by the diaphragm.

C. It continues inferiorly into the pelvic cavity. The two continuous cavities are sometimes referred to as the abdominopelvic cavity.

D. The abdominal cavity is divided into four quadrants by the transverse line and the midline.

E. Organs

   1. Esophagus: collapsible digestive structure running from mouth to stomach. The esophagus resides posterior to the trachea.

   2. Stomach: hollow digestive organ in LUQ. The stomach receives food, begins breaking it down, and sends it to the small intestine.

   3. Pancreas: solid organ that aids in digestion, produces insulin, and helps regulate blood glucose levels.

   4. Liver: solid organ; occupies most of the RUQ. The liver helps break down fats, filters toxins, and produces cholesterol.

   5. Gallbladder: a hollow organ positioned beneath the liver. The gallbladder collects and stores bile from the liver. It releases bile into the intestine to aid in digestion.

6. Small intestine: hollow organ that occupies both lower abdominal quadrants. Food from the stomach is mixed with digestive enzymes to digest fat. Most of the contents are absorbed out of the small intestine and used or stored by the body.

7. Large intestine: hollow organ that includes the colon and rectum. Occupies the outer border of the abdomen. The large intestine pulls most of the remaining liquid to form solid stool.

8. Appendix: a hollow organ in the RLQ. It can become easily obstructed, causing inflammation, rupture, and life-threatening infection.

9. Spleen: a solid organ with little protection in the LUQ. The spleen filters the blood. It has a rich blood supply and can be a source of severe internal bleeding.

10. Kidneys: solid organs that are part of the urinary system. The kidneys control fluid balance, filter waste, and control pH balance.

 XII. ENDOCRINE SYSTEM

A. A system of glands that secrete hormones into the blood to help regulate body functions

B. Responsible for insulin production and regulation of blood glucose levels

 XIII. URINARY SYSTEM

A. Filters waste from the blood through the kidneys

B. Controls fluid balance in the body

C. Controls pH (acid-base balance) to maintain homeostasis

D. Ureters are tubes connecting each kidney to the bladder. Urine moves from the kidneys through the ureters into the bladder and then through the urethra and out of the body.

XIV. REPRODUCTIVE SYSTEM

A. Males: includes testicles, penis, and sperm. The prostate gland is part of the male reproductive system. It surrounds the urethra near the bladder.

B. Females: includes ovaries, fallopian tubes, and vagina.

XV. CELLULAR ENERGY AND METABOLISM

A. Adenosine Triphosphate (ATP)

1. The body uses oxygen to convert nutrients into cellular energy called ATP.

2. Cells receive exponentially more ATP if there is an adequate oxygen supply.

B. Aerobic Metabolism

1. Aerobic metabolism is the creation of cellular energy with the use of oxygen. It is by far the most efficient means of energy production.

2. The heart and brain will cease function without an adequate supply of oxygen. The lungs and kidneys are also very sensitive to a lack of oxygen.

3. The waste products of aerobic metabolism are water and carbon dioxide. The human body is well equipped to handle these by-products through the respiratory and urinary systems.

C. Anaerobic Metabolism

1. Anaerobic metabolism is the creation of energy without an adequate oxygen supply. Much of the body (not the heart or brain) can switch over to an anaerobic metabolism when necessary.

2. The body will triage the oxygen supply when necessary, sending it to the most critical areas and forcing other areas into an anaerobic state.

3. The by-products of anaerobic metabolism include lactic acid. The body needs much longer to deal with by-products of anaerobic metabolism and cannot complete the process until adequate oxygen supply is restored.

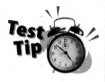

Compared to the previous EMT training curriculum, the current National EMS Education Standards place a stronger emphasis on anatomy, physiology, pathophysiology, and terminology. This emphasis will definitely be reflected on the national certification exam. Be sure to study the material in this chapter.

XVI. INFANTS AND CHILDREN

A. Anatomical Differences from Adults

1. The pediatric tongue is larger in proportion to the airway.

2. The pediatric airway is more easily obstructed.

3. The pediatric head is larger in proportion to the body.

Author's Note: The internet is replete with illustrations of the anatomical structures and systems presented in this chapter. If you are struggling with any of the information presented in this chapter, I recommend you do an internet search for "images of . . . ."

PRACTICE QUESTIONS
Answers on page 381.

1. Movement of air in and out of the lungs is called

   A. cellular respiration.

   B. external respiration.

   C. internal respiration.

   D. pulmonary ventilation.

2. The frontal plane divides the body into
   A. left and right sides.
   B. top and bottom halves.
   C. anterior and posterior.
   D. proximal and distal.

3. From the anatomical position, which of the following is the lateral bone in the forearm?
   A. the ulna
   B. the radius
   C. the humerus
   D. the tibia

4. Which of the following are true regarding pediatric patients? (Select the THREE answer options that apply.)
   A. The pediatric tongue is larger in proportion to the airway.
   B. The pediatric tongue takes up very little space in the upper airway.
   C. The structure of the pediatric airway makes airway obstruction unlikely.
   D. The pediatric airway is more easily obstructed.
   E. The pediatric head is larger in proportion to the body.
   F. The pediatric head is smaller in proportion to the body.

5. Your patient is experiencing inadequate tissue perfusion. This is known as
   A. shock.
   B. hypoxia.
   C. anemia.
   D. hypotension.

Life Span Development

I. **TERMS TO KNOW**

A. **Fontanelles:** Soft spots in the newborn/infant's skull.

B. **Infant:** Up to one year of age.

C. **Neonate:** Newborn from birth to 28 days of age.

D. **Preschooler:** 3 to 6 years of age.

E. **Toddler:** One to 3 years of age.

I. **INFANTS**

A. Ages

1. Neonate: a newborn from birth to one month of age

2. Infant: up to one year of age

B. Vital Signs

1. Respirations. Normal respiratory rate is about 30 to 60 breaths per minute (bpm) for newborns and about 25 to 50 bpm for infants.

2. Pulse. Normal pulse rate is about 140 to 160 beats per minute for newborns and about 100 to 140 beats per minute for infants.

3. Blood pressure. A newborn's blood pressure is about 70 systolic and will increase to about 90 systolic by one year of age.

C. Physiology

1. The typical newborn weight is about 6 to 8 pounds (3 to 3.5 kilograms). The newborn's weight will typically double by six months and triple by about one year.

2. The newborn's head makes up about 25% of the body and is a significant source of heat loss.

3. During the first couple weeks, neonates often lose weight, and then begin to gain it back.

4. The newborn's fontanelles will usually be fully fused by about 18 months. Depressed fontanelles may indicate hypovolemia. Bulging fontanelles indicate increased pressure within the skull.

5. Infants are often nose breathers and can develop respiratory distress easily.

6. Rapid breathing can lead to fluid loss and loss of body heat.

7. Hyperventilation of infants presents significant risk of barotrauma.

D. Neonates typically have

1. startle reflex: open arms wide, spreading fingers

2. grip reflex: grip when something placed in palm

3. rooting reflex: turn toward a touch to the cheek

4. sucking reflex: stimulated by touching the lips

E. Infants

1. At 6 months: typically begin teething, can sit upright, and track objects visually

2. At 12 months

    i. Typically know their name, recognize parents or caregivers, walk with assistance, and speak a few words

    ii. Still communicate distress primarily through crying

II. TODDLERS AND PRESCHOOLERS

A. Age

1. Toddlers: one to 3 years old

2. Preschoolers: 3 to 6 years old

B. Vitals

    1. Toddlers

        i. Respirations: about 20 to 30 bpm

        ii. Heart rate: about 90 to 140 beats per minute

        iii. Blood pressure: about 80 to 90 systolic

    2. Preschoolers

        i. Respirations: about 20 to 25 bpm

        ii. Heart rate: 80 to 130 beats per minute

        iii. Blood pressure: about 90 to 110 systolic

C. Physiology

    1. As the immune system develops, children at this age typically experience a number of minor colds, viruses, flu-like symptoms, respiratory infections, etc.

    2. Fine motor skills improve, and the brain grows rapidly in size.

D. Toddlers typically walk, climb, distinguish basic shapes and colors, and are potty trained.

E. Preschoolers typically

    1. are physically coordinated and communicate well verbally

    2. know their name and address and can dress themselves

    3. can count to 10 or beyond

F. Recommendations

    1. Separation anxiety is common. Allow child to stay with caregiver when possible.

    2. Communicate directly with the child, not just the caregivers.

    3. Choose your words carefully. They will probably be taken literally.

    4. Do not lie.

SCHOOL-AGE CHILDREN: 6 TO 12 YEARS OLD

A. Vitals

    1. Respirations: about 15 to 20 bpm

    2. Heart rate: 70 to 110 beats per minute

    3. Blood pressure: about 90 to 120 systolic

B. Physiology

    1. Permanent teeth replace baby teeth.

    2. The musculoskeletal system is growing rapidly.

C. School-age children typically

    1. read and write

    2. develop basic problem-solving skills

    3. are establishing their self-image and morals

    4. have a large social circle due to school

    5. understand the concept of death

    6. look up to authority figures such as police officers and firefighters

D. Recommendations

    1. Communicate in understandable terms, but do not talk down to them.

    2. Respect the privacy rights for this age group.

 ADOLESCENTS: 12 TO 18 YEARS OF AGE

A. Vitals

    1. Respirations: 12 to 20 bpm

    2. Heart rate: 60 to 100 beats per minute

    3. Blood pressure: about 100 to 120 systolic

B. Physiology

1. Significant physical growth occurs over about a three-year period.

2. Eating disorders are most common in adolescents and young adults up to age 25. They are also much more common in females.

3. Puberty occurs.

C. Adolescents often

1. exhibit argumentative behavior, and are hypercritical and egocentric

2. do not anticipate the consequences of their actions

3. are subject to a great deal of peer pressure, and are at higher risk for depression and suicide

4. are preoccupied with body image and physical appearance

5. become sexually active

D. Recommendation: For sensitive matters, talk with the adolescent without caregivers present when possible.

 V. ADULTHOOD

A. Stages of Adulthood

1. Early adulthood: 20 to 40 years of age

2. Middle adulthood: 40 to 60 years of age

3. Late adulthood: over 60 years of age

B. Vitals

1. Respirations: 12 to 20 bpm

2. Heart rate: 60 to 100 beats per minute

3. Blood pressure: about 110/70 to 130/90

C. Characteristics

1. Accidental trauma is a leading cause of death in the young adult age group.

2. Mild physical decline typically develops in the middle-adult age group.

3. Women typically experience menopause during middle adulthood.

4. Continued physical and mental decline is common in late adulthood.

5. Older adults frequently have extensive medical histories and are on multiple medications.

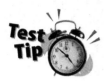
Test Tip

Priority-of-treatment questions are common on the certification exam. These questions are often scenario-based and end with, "Your next action should be . . ." or, "Your first action should be . . ."

Such questions test your patient assessment knowledge. Patient assessment isn't a category on the certification exam, it's *every* category on the certification exam.

PRACTICE QUESTIONS
Answers on page 382.

1. While assessing an infant, you note depressed fontanelles. This most likely indicates that the infant

   A. is dehydrated.

   B. is perfusing normally.

   C. has brain swelling.

   D. has been crying recently.

2. Your patient is 2 years old. She would be considered a(n)

   A. neonate.

   B. infant.

   C. toddler.

   D. preschooler.

3. To ease a child's anxiety, it is usually best to

    A. isolate the child.

    B. avoid eye contact.

    C. keep caregivers close by.

    D. place the child supine.

4. Eating disorders are more common among which of the following age groups?

    A. adolescents

    B. school-age

    C. toddlers

    D. older adults

5. Which of the following statements is correct? (Select the TWO answer options that apply.)

    A. Physical decline typically begins in the young adult age group.

    B. Women usually develop menopause during early adulthood.

    C. Older adults are likely on multiple medications.

    D. Accidental trauma is the leading cause of death in young adults.

    E. Middle adults typically do not anticipate the consequences of their actions.

PART III

ASSESSMENT, AIRWAY, RESPIRATION, AND VENTILATION

REVIEW PLUS
END-OF-CHAPTER PRACTICE

History Taking, Vital Signs, and Monitoring Devices

I. TERMS TO KNOW

A. **Associated symptoms:** Anything the patient complains of in addition to the chief complaint.

B. **Glucometry:** Assessment of blood glucose levels.

C. **Pertinent negatives:** Anything relevant to the chief complaint that the patient denies.

D. **Pulse pressure:** The difference between systolic and diastolic pressures.

E. **Trending:** Routine monitoring and reassessment to identify changes.

II. HISTORY TAKING

A. Chief Complaint

   1. The chief complaint is the patient's primary reason for calling EMS.

   2. The patient history will generally begin by determining the chief complaint.

   3. If unable to determine the chief complaint from the patient, question family, bystanders, etc.

   4. Other EMS providers can simultaneously begin other assessments or interventions as resources and the patient's condition allow.

B. History of Present Illness (HPI)

   1. Once the chief complaint has been established, begin obtaining the HPI.

2. The HPI includes:

    i.   Basic patient information, such as age, sex, weight

    ii.   Additional information about the chief complaint

    iii.   Associated signs and symptoms

    iv.   General health status

    v.   Past medical history

    vi.   Medications

    vii.   Allergies

C. Techniques for History Taking

1. Take notes to ensure accuracy.

2. Open-ended questions

    i.   Open-ended questions require a descriptive response, not just a "yes" or "no."

    ii.   Preferred when you want the patients to describe things in their own words.

    iii.   These questions take longer to answer but provide more information from the patient's perspective. Examples:

       ➤ "Why did you call for help today?"

       ➤ "How would you describe the pain?"

       ➤ "What were you doing when this started?"

3. Closed questions

    i.   Closed questions can be answered quickly with a "yes" or "no" response (verbally or nonverbally).

    ii.   Preferred when time is short. Example: "Are you choking?" is more appropriate than "Can you describe how it feels to be choking?"

    iii.   Useful when patient is unable to speak without difficulty, such as airway obstruction, severe pain, or respiratory distress.

    iv.   These questions elicit faster responses but lead to answers that are less descriptive.

4. Active listening techniques

    i.   Try to have one provider obtain the patient history. If several people are directing questions to the patient, it is harder to establish a rapport and stay organized.

    ii.   Face the patient, maintain eye contact, and show that you are listening.

    iii.   Repeating what the patient has said demonstrates you are listening and may elicit additional information.

    iv.   Do not interrupt the patient.

    v.   Clarify vague or unclear statements.

    vi.   Your questions should not be biased or judgmental.

    vii.   Show empathy, such as, "I can understand why you feel that way."

    viii.   Be alert for contradictions or unclear information. For example, the patient states he has no medical history, but is on prescription medications. Patients will often state that they are allergic to a medication but describe common side effects of the medication.

    ix.   Ask the most important questions first. Have an organized approach but allow flexibility. For example, questioning your trauma patient about neck pain would be a higher priority than asking about medical history.

D. Aids to History Taking

1. SAMPLE history (a mnemonic for remembering the questions to ask during assessment of the patient).

    i.   Signs and symptoms

       ➤ Signs are findings you can objectively see, feel, hear, or smell. Examples: vomiting, deformity, wheezing.

       ➤ Symptoms are subjective feelings that the patient must tell you about. Examples: nausea, pain, dyspnea.

    ii.   Allergies: any allergies to medications, including prescription (Rx) and over-the-counter (OTC) meds.

    iii.   Medications

       ➤ Any medications the patient takes regularly, including Rx and OTC, vitamins, herbals, supplements, etc.

➤ Any medications taken recently

➤ Any illicit drugs

➤ Marijuana, tobacco, vapes

➤ Any medications for erectile dysfunction (especially important for a cardiac patient who may be a candidate for nitroglycerin)

➤ Be sure to spell the medications correctly and include the dose and frequency.

> *Note:* Most elderly patients are prescribed at least four different medications (polypharmacy: the simultaneous use of multiple medications by one person).

  iv. Past pertinent history

➤ Any relevant past medical history

➤ Any condition the patient takes medication to treat

➤ Any history similar to the current chief complaint

  v. Last oral intake

➤ Most recent food and fluid intake

➤ May be important for surgical candidates, diabetics, any patient at risk for vomiting

  vi. Events leading to incident

➤ What events led up to the chief complaint?

➤ Anything unusual, e.g., activities, food, new medications, recent injury, travel, etc.

2. OPQRST

  i. OPQRST is used to assess the patient's symptoms, especially pain, but it can be adapted to other chief complaints, such as dizziness.

  ii. **O**nset: "What were you doing when the pain/symptom began?"

  iii. **P**rovocation: "Does anything make your pain/symptom better or worse?"

iv. **Quality:** "How would you describe the pain/symptom?"

v. **Radiation:** "Does the pain move, or go anywhere?"

vi. **Severity:** "How would you rate the pain on a scale from 0 to 10, with 10 being the most severe?"

vii. **Time:** "When did the pain/symptom begin?"

3. Associated symptoms and pertinent negatives

   i. Associated symptoms: anything the patient complains of in addition to the chief complaint.

   ii. Pertinent negatives: anything relevant to the chief complaint that the patient denies.

   iii. Examples:

   ➤ You should always ask a chest pain patient if they are also having dyspnea. If they are, then dyspnea is an associated symptom. If the patient denies dyspnea, then it is a pertinent negative.

   ➤ You should always ask your trauma patient if they have neck pain, in addition to their chief complaint. If yes, then it is an associated symptom. If the patient denies neck pain, then it is a pertinent negative.

4. Special situations

   i. At times, it will be necessary to ask the patient about sensitive topics, such as assault, drug use, erectile dysfunction medications, possible pregnancy, etc.

   ➤ Limit your questions to those that are necessary and relevant.

   ➤ Be direct, professional, and non-judgmental.

   ➤ Provide as much privacy as possible.

   ii. At times, gathering a patient history can be unusually challenging. Use your active listening techniques and remain professional. Challenging situations may include:

   ➤ Patients under the influence of alcohol or drugs

   ➤ Victims of assault or abuse

   ➤ Non-communicative or overly talkative patients

➤ Patients with multiple complaints

➤ Anxious, frightened, or emotional patients

➤ Patients with cognitive disabilities

➤ Patients with behavioral problems

➤ Hostile or threatening patients

➤ Pediatric patients

II. VITAL SIGNS

A. Vital signs ("vitals") provide a combination of quantitative (numerical) and qualitative (non-numerical) data. This data is used to establish a baseline and monitor for changes over time. Every patient encounter should include at least two sets of vital signs and continued monitoring over time. If, for some reason, this is not done, your PCR should indicate why.

   i.   "Baseline" vitals are the first set taken.

   ii. "Trending" vitals refer to the reassessment and comparison of vitals over time. This can help identify improvement or deterioration in the patient's condition.

   iii. Stable patients: Reassess vitals every 15 minutes.

   iv. Unstable patients: Reassess vitals every 5 minutes.

B. The list of what is considered a "vital sign" is growing as patient care and patient monitoring devices evolves.

   1. The six standard vital signs

      i.   Respirations

      ii. Pulse

      iii. Blood pressure

      iv. Pupils

      v.   Skin / temperature

      vi. Pulse oximetry

   2. Additional patient monitoring used by EMTs

      i.   Blood glucose monitoring

      ii. Glasgow Coma Scale

C. Respirations: rate, rhythm, and quality

1. Usually assessed by observing the patient's chest rise and fall. Sometimes it's easier to feel respirations by placing a hand on the chest or auscultate (listen) to respirations with a stethoscope.

2. Respiratory rate: Breaths per minute. Count the number of breaths (inhalation **or** exhalation, not both) for 30 seconds and double it for the rate per minute.

   i. Normal respiratory rates

      ➤ Adult: 12 to 20 breaths per minute

      ➤ Children (school-age): 18 to 30 breaths per minute

      ➤ Toddlers: 24 to 40 breaths per minute

      ➤ Infants: 30 to 60 breaths per minute

   ii. Abnormal respiratory rates

      ➤ Tachypnea: rapid breathing (over 20 breaths per minute in an adult)

      ➤ Bradypnea: slow breathing (under 12 breaths per minute)

   iii. Respiratory rhythm and tidal volume

      ➤ Normal: regular rhythm and adequate chest rise and fall

      ➤ Shallow: minimal chest rise and fall

      ➤ Labored: increased work of breathing

      ➤ Irregular: abnormal breathing pattern

3. Tidal volume and minute volume

   i. Tidal volume: The amount of air that moves in or out of the lungs with each breath. Normal tidal volume for an adult is 400 to 500 mL.

   ii. Minute volume: Also called minute ventilation. Minute ventilation = tidal volume × respiratory rate. Example: If the respiratory rate is 12 and the tidal volume is 400 mL, then the minute volume is 4,800 mL.

   iii. Documentation of respirations

      ➤ Always document both rate and quality of respirations.

      ➤ Example: "16 & normal," "24 & shallow," "40 & labored"

    iv. Auscultation of lung sounds

➤ Some consider auscultation of lung sounds part of the respiratory component of vital signs. Others consider lung sounds part of the physical exam.

➤ Lung sounds are usually heard better from the patient's back, not the anterior chest.

— Normal: clear lung sounds in both left and right lungs ("clear and equal bilaterally")

— Wheezing: high-pitched whistling sound, typically more noticeable on expiration

— Crackles/Rales: wet, crackling sounds, usually on inspiration and expiration

— Rhonchi: low-pitched, congested sounds often due to mucus in the lungs, usually on expiration

➤ Auscultate lung sounds under clothing in three fields:

— Upper lungs (apices): below the clavicles, midclavicular line

— Middle lung field: middle chest, midclavicular, posterior

— Lower lungs (base): lower portion of thorax, midclavicular or midaxillary

D. Pulse: rate, rhythm, quality (e.g., 70, strong, regular)

  1. It is unlikely that you will be able to palpate a pulse if the patient's blood pressure is below 60 mmHg systolic.

  2. Pulse checks for unresponsive patients that may be in cardiac arrest

    i. Adults and children: carotid pulse

    ii. Infants: brachial pulse

  3. Pulse checks for conscious patients (CPR not needed)

    i. Adults and children: radial pulse

    ii. Infants: brachial pulse

  4. Pulse rate: count the pulse rate for 30 seconds and double it for the beats per minute.

    i. Normal pulse rates

➤ Adults: 60 to 100 beats per minute

➤ Children: 80 to 120 beats per minute

➤ Infants: 100 to 180 beats per minute

    ii.   Abnormal pulse rates

➤ Tachycardia: rapid pulse (over 100 beats per minute)

➤ Bradycardia: slow pulse (under 60 beats per minute)

    iii. Pulse quality and rhythm

➤ Quality: strong or weak

➤ Rhythm: regular or irregular

5. Documentation of pulse

    i.   Always document rate, rhythm, and quality of pulses

    ii.   Example: "82 strong and regular," "100 weak and irregular"

E. Blood pressure (BP)

1. Blood pressure measures the pressure exerted against the arteries during contraction of the left ventricle (systole) and in between contractions of the left ventricle (diastole).

2. BP is measured in millimeters of mercury (mmHg) with a sphygmomanometer (BP cuff) and a stethoscope or an automated non-invasive BP (NIBP) monitoring device.

3. Sample BP: 130/80

    i.   Systolic BP: the top number. Systole represents the pressure within the arteries during contraction of the heart.

    ii.   Diastolic BP: the bottom number. Diastole represents the pressure within the arteries between cardiac contractions. Diastolic pressure is always lower than systolic pressure.

    iii. Manual BP readings should be documented in even numbers. NIBP can provide odd numbers.

    iv. Pulse pressure

➤ The difference between systolic and diastolic pressures. Example: If the patient's BP is 130/80, then the pulse pressure is 50.

➤ Normal pulse pressure: greater than 25% but less than 50% of systolic pressure.

➤ Wide pulse pressure: pulse pressure above 50% of systolic pressure. Indicates increased pressure within the brain. Example: 210/100 (pulse pressure is 110).

➤ Narrow pulse pressure: pulse pressure below 25% of systolic pressure. Indicates possible obstructive shock (tension pneumothorax, cardiac tamponade, pulmonary embolism).

4. Blood pressure values

   i. Adults

   ➤ Normal: below 120/80 (systolic must be below 120 **and** diastolic must be below 80)

   ➤ Elevated: 120 to 129/less than 80

   ➤ Stage 1 hypertension: 130 to 139/80 to 89

   ➤ Stage 2 hypertension: systolic 140 or above **or** diastolic 90 or higher

   ➤ Hypertensive crisis: systolic above 180 and/or diastolic above 120

   ii. Children

   ➤ Ages one to 10 years

   — Normal: 80 + 2(age)/two-thirds systolic. Example: 5-year-old patient: 90/60.

   — Hypotension: systolic below 70 + 2(age). Example: a 5-year-old with a systolic BP below 80 requires further evaluation for possible shock.

5. Blood pressure by palpation

   i. BP by palpation (feel) does not require a stethoscope but it only provides a systolic pressure.

   ii. BP by palpation is less accurate and is **never** preferred to BP by auscultation (listening). It may be necessary , however, if unable to hear due to environment or equipment issues.

6. Orthostatic hypotension (aka postural hypotension)

   i. Assess patient's BP and pulse while supine. Patient should be supine for about 5 minutes before assessing BP and pulse.

   ii. Have the patient stand for 1 minute and repeat BP and pulse.

    iii. A drop in systolic BP above 20 mmHg or a drop in diastolic BP above 10 mmHg is considered abnormal.

    iv. A sharp rise in pulse rate when the patient stands may indicate the body is attempting to compensate for falling BP.

    v. Abnormal findings may indicate hypovolemia or increased risk of syncope and fall injury.

    vi. Do **not** assess for orthostatic hypotension if the patient is already dizzy, weak, or hypotensive while supine. Follow local protocols.

F. Pupils: size, equality, shape, reactivity

  1. Size

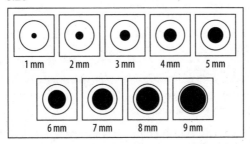

    i. Assess the pupil (dark center) of both eyes.

    ii. Midsize: normal (2 to 5 mm in light)

    iii. Dilated: large "mydriasis"

    iv. Constricted: small "miosis"

  2. Equality

    i. Equal: both pupils are round and equal.

    ii. Unequal: pupils are different size or shape (anisocoria).

  3. Reactivity

    i. Pupils should constrict (get smaller) in response to light and dilate (get larger) in the dark. *Note:* Pupils constrict, they don't "contract."

    ii. Pupillary constriction should be rapid, not sluggish.

    iii. Attempting to assess pupillary constriction with a penlight in a bright environment (outdoors) will likely be ineffective.

iv. "Fixed and dilated" refers to pupils that are large and non-reactive to light. This indicates probable severe injury or illness.

4. Documenting. There are several ways to document pupils:

    i. PEARL: pupils equal and reactive to light.

    ii. PERRL: pupils equal, round, and reactive to light.

    iii. "Pupils midpoint, equal, and reactive."

G. Skin: color, temperature, condition/moisture, capillary refill

1. The skin provides clues to how well the respiratory and circulatory systems are functioning.

2. Skin color

    i. Check skin color by looking at the nail beds, palms of the hands, or soles of the feet.

    ii. Abnormal findings

        ➤ Pale: also called pallor. May indicate lack of blood flow due to poor circulation.

        ➤ Cyanosis: bluish color. May indicate a lack of oxygen.

        ➤ Flushed: red skin. May indicate excessive heat, fever, exertion.

        ➤ Jaundice: yellow skin. May indicate liver disease.

        ➤ Mottling: a "marbled" or "patchy" appearance to the skin, often with red or purple. Indicates a lack of blood flow.

3. Temperature

    i. Normal temperatures:

        ➤ Average body temperature is 98.6° F (37° C), but normal range is 97° F (36.1° C) to 99° F (37.2° C).

        ➤ Elderly patients often have lower body temperatures.

    ii. Fever: the following generally indicate a fever

        ➤ Rectal, ear, or temporal: 100.4° (38° C) or higher.

        ➤ Oral: 100° F (37.8° C) or higher.

        ➤ Axillary (armpit): 99° F (37.2° C) or higher.

Note: When treating a patient with a fever, consider the severity and possible causes of the fever. Generally, treatment should focus on relieving discomfort, promoting rest, and hydration. Treating the fever does not shorten the course of illness.

    iii.   Relative skin temperature

- To assess relative skin temperature, palpate the patient's skin on the upper back or neck (not the forehead) using the back of your hand.

- Assessing relative skin temperature is less exact, but faster, than using a thermometer. It can provide quick, qualitative information, e.g., "hot" or "cold."

4. Condition

    i.   Dry: normal (not excessively dry)

    ii.   Wet: excessive sweating, also called "diaphoretic." Abnormal. Causes include menopause, diabetes, cardiac emergency, anaphylaxis, drug/alcohol withdrawal.

    iii.   Clammy: cool and moist. Abnormal. May indicate shock.

5. Capillary refill

    i.   Capillary refill is a measurement of how long it takes for capillaries to refill after being squeezed.

    ii.   Capillary refill is used in pediatric patients (under about 6 years) to assess for possible signs of poor perfusion. Capillary refill is *not* a reliable indicator of perfusion in adults.

    iii.   Compress the nailbed until it blanches (whitens). Release and count the number of seconds it takes to return to normal.

- Normal capillary refill: 2 seconds or less.

- Delayed capillary refill: more than 2 seconds. Indicates the need for further assessment for possible shock.

6. Documenting skin findings

    i.   Example: "Skin warm, pink, dry"

    ii.   Example: "Skin warm, dry, 98.7° F"

    iii.   Example: "Skin pale, cool, clammy, capillary refill 3 seconds"

III. PATIENT MONITORING DEVICES

A. Here are a few common patient monitoring devices EMTs will use or assist with:

1. Blood glucose monitoring

2. Pulse oximetry

3. Non-invasive blood pressure monitoring

4. Capnography

B. Blood glucose monitoring

1. Glucometers are used to test the blood sugar levels in the capillaries or veins.

2. Glucometers that are maintained and used properly provide blood glucose levels that are nearly as accurate as a lab.

3. Glucometers used in the prehospital setting require a blood sample and do not provide continuous monitoring of blood glucose levels.

4. Many diabetic patients today have app-based smart glucometers that provide continuous monitoring of blood glucose levels. Smart glucometers will connect to a smart phone or watch. They also do not require finger sticks.

5. Blood glucose levels

   i. Normal: between 80 and 120 mg/dL (4.4 to 6.7 mmol/L)

   ii Hypoglycemia: low blood glucose

   iii. Hyperglycemia: high blood glucose

6. Indications for blood glucose testing

   i. Any patient with an altered level of consciousness

   ii. Any patient with a known or suspected diabetic problem

C. Pulse oximetry

1. Pulse oximeters provide a non-invasive method of measuring the saturation of oxygen in the blood. They help assess the patient's respiratory efficiency and need for supplemental oxygen.

2. Pulse oximetry (SaO_2) is part of the standard of care in EMS today and is considered a vital sign. You should assess SaO_2 levels on any patient who you collect vital signs on.

3. A normal SaO_2 is 94% to 99% (or 95% to 100%, depending on the source).

4. Limitations of pulse oximetry

   i.   Pulse oximetry is one assessment tool for respiratory efficiency, not the only tool.

   ii. Pulse oximeters cannot measure the amount of hemoglobin, only the oxygen saturation of the hemoglobin that is present.

   iii. Inaccurate readings may be caused by hypovolemia, hypothermia, anemia, nail polish, carbon monoxide poisoning, and tobacco use.

D. Non-invasive blood pressure monitoring (NIBP)

   1. Most cardiac monitors used in EMS today perform several functions, including automatic blood pressure readings that don't require auscultation with a stethoscope.

   2. If the NIBP reading does not match the patient's clinical presentation, you should manually assess the patient's BP by auscultation.

E. Capnography

   1. Capnography is the measurement of carbon dioxide in the patient's exhaled breath.

   2. Also called end-tidal CO_2 ($ETCO_2$) monitoring. It provides information about the patient's ventilation and perfusion status.

   3. Capnography displays a CO_2 waveform and a numerical value, while capnometry only provides a numerical value.

   4. In some EMS systems, EMTs may assist advanced-level providers with the equipment setup for capnography or capnometry (follow local protocol). Interpretation of capnography is considered an advanced skill (AEMT or paramedic).

PRACTICE QUESTIONS
Answers on page 383.

1. Your elderly patient takes five prescription medications. This is known as
   A. multimeds.
   B. polypharmacy.
   C. drug dependency.
   D. co-pharmacy.

2. While supine, your patient's blood pressure was 134/90. You reassessed the patient's blood pressure while he was standing and it dropped to 100/78. This is known as
   A. orthostatic hypotension.
   B. standing hypertension.
   C. orthopnea.
   D. vertical hypotension.

3. Which of the following blood glucose levels is considered normal?
   A. 400 mg/dL
   B. 200 mg/dL
   C. 100 mg/dL
   D. 50 mg/dL

4. Which of the following statements are correct? (Select the TWO correct answer options that apply.)
   A. Cyanosis indicates a lack of oxygen.
   B. Pale indicates a lack of vitamin D.
   C. Flushed indicates a lack of blood flow.
   D. Jaundiced indicates liver problems.
   E. Mottling indicates normal circulation.

5. Your 5-year-old patient is unresponsive. To determine whether CPR is needed, you should immediately assess the

A. radial pulse.

B. brachial pulse.

C. carotid pulse.

D. pedal pulse.

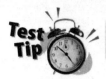

Test Tip

A multiple-choice question that requires more than one answer is called a multiple-response question. You may see a number of such questions on the national certification exam.

Patient Assessment

TERMS TO KNOW

A. **Baseline vitals:** The first set of vitals.

B. **Flail chest:** Two or more contiguous rib fractures with two or more breaks per rib.

C. **Mechanism of injury (MOI):** The type of injury that occurred.

D. **Nature of illness (NOI):** The nature of the medical complaint.

E. **Sucking chest wound:** Penetrating thoracic wound that allows air into the pleural space.

THE FIVE COMPONENTS OF PATIENT ASSESSMENT FOR EMTS

A. Scene size-up

B. Primary assessment

C. Patient history

D. Secondary assessment

E. Reassessment

III. **SCENE SIZE-UP**

A. Begins as soon as the call is received and doesn't end until the call is over

B. Scene safety

1. Your safety is your first priority. If the scene is safe, continue with your assessment. If it is not safe, either make it safe or leave immediately and request assistance.

2. Rescuers are required to wear an approved high-visibility safety vest at all accident scenes or anytime working near traffic.

3. A portable, impact-resistant, high-intensity flashlight should be carried at all times.

4. Keep your portable radio and cellphone with you whenever possible.

5. Position your emergency vehicle for easy access and to protect the scene if necessary. **Never** position the loading compartment of the ambulance in the path of oncoming traffic.

6. Some EMS systems will dispatch rescuers to a potentially dangerous scene that has not yet been secured by law enforcement, but will be told to "stage." Staging means you remain a safe distance from the scene until cleared by law enforcement.

C. Standard Precautions

1. Take standard precautions and utilize appropriate PPE.

2. The level of PPE required will vary depending on the nature of the call.

D. Number of patients / additional resources

1. Determine the number of patients.

2. Request additional resources as needed (advanced life support, additional ambulances, extrication, law enforcement, etc.).

E. Mechanism of injury / nature of illness

1. The patient is usually the best source of information; however, at times it will be necessary to question family members or bystanders.

2. Mechanism of injury (MOI)

   i. MOI is for trauma patients.

   ii. What type of trauma occurred (fall injury, vehicle accident, assault, etc.)?

   iii. Understanding the MOI can help predict injury patterns, influence treatment decisions, and help determine hospital destination.

3. Nature of illness (NOI)

   i. NOI is for medical patients.

   ii. What is the nature of the complaint (respiratory, cardiac, behavioral, etc.)?

   iii. The NOI will be related to the patient's chief complaint, but it is not the same thing. For example, the patient could have a chief complaint of chest pain, but it could be due to a respiratory problem or a traumatic injury.

4. Patients may experience both a medical condition and traumatic injury, e.g., a fall injury due to syncope, or a motor vehicle collision due to a seizure.

F. Consider spinal precautions

1. Based on the information obtained, consider the possible need for spinal precautions.

2. Follow local protocols regarding spinal precautions.

3. The term "spinal immobilization" and associated interventions are no longer part of the national curriculum. Spinal precautions, when needed, are now referred to as "spinal motion restriction." See Chapter 18 for more information on management of spinal injuries.

IV. PRIMARY ASSESSMENT

A. The primary assessment begins as soon as you reach the patient. Remember, the scene size-up doesn't end. You are continuously monitoring and ensuring scene safety, maintaining appropriate PPE, etc.

B. The purpose of the primary assessment is to identify and manage life-threatening conditions.

C. General impression

    1. The general impression is based on the information you can gather immediately upon arrival at the patient.

    2. Use all relevant senses to form a general impression. Consider the patient's approximate age, gender, level of distress, overall appearance, etc.

D. Level of consciousness (LOC)

    1. During the primary assessment, the first assessment of LOC is general, not specific. Determine whether the patient is . . .

        i.   Conscious and alert, or

        ii.   Conscious and altered, or

        iii. Unconscious

    2. AVPU scale is used to rapidly determine the patient's general responsiveness

        i.   A = Awake, e.g., patient's eyes are open and tracking you.

        ii.   V = Responsive to voice, e.g., "Hey, are you OK?!"

        iii. P = Responsive to pain.

        iv. U = Unconscious/unresponsive.

    3. Person, place, time, event (A&Ox4)

        i.   If your patient is awake and there are no obvious life threats, you can begin a more in-depth assessment of the patient's mentation (alertness and orientation to surroundings).

            ➤ Person: Does the patient know his or her name?

            ➤ Place: Does the patient know where he or she is?

            ➤ Time: Does the patient know the year, month, and approximate date and time?

            ➤ Event: Can the patient describe the current MOI or NOI?

        ii.   Patients that are oriented to person, place, time, and event are referred to as "A&Ox4." If the patient has trouble with one of these assessments, they are referred to as "A&Ox3."

4. When dealing with unconscious patients (CAB assessment—circulation, airway, breathing) . . .

   i. Remember, conscious patients do *not* need CPR; however, unconscious patients *may* need CPR. Current American Heart Association guidelines recommend checking for a pulse for 5 to 10 seconds on unresponsive patients to determine whether CPR is needed.

   ii. When an unresponsive patient does need CPR, you should initiate chest compressions immediately after determining pulselessness.

   iii. For these reasons, you should conduct your primary assessment for unresponsive patients using the Circulation, Airway, Breathing (CAB) approach.

   iv. The CAB approach is also indicated if your patient has obvious life-threatening external bleeding.

   v. Patients who are *not* unconscious (and therefore obviously don't need CPR) and without severe bleeding should be assessed using the traditional Airway, Breathing, Circulation (ABC) approach.

Note: You **must** assess LOC to determine if your primary assessment will follow the ABC approach or the CAB approach. Unconscious or severe bleeding = CAB. Everyone else = ABC. This is a critical concept!

V. **AIRWAY** (see Chapter 10 for more detailed information)

A. Assess the airway and intervene as needed. A *patent* airway means the patient's airway is clear and is not obstructing breathing.

B. The patient's LOC is a key factor in determining what airway interventions are needed. Do *not* assume that patients with a decreased LOC are able to adequately protect their own airway.

C. The three key steps in airway

   1. Manual airway maneuvers (as needed)

      i. Head-tilt, chin-lift (no spinal injury suspected)

      ii. Jaw thrust maneuvers (suspected spinal cord injury)

2. Suction the upper airway (as needed)

3. Mechanical airway adjunct (as needed)

    i. Oropharyngeal airway (OPA): unresponsive patients with no gag reflex only.

    ii. Nasopharyngeal airway (NPA): patients with decreased LOC.

 VI. BREATHING (see Chapter 10 for more detailed information.)

A. Assess respiratory rate, rhythm, and quality and auscultate lung sounds (see Chapter 10 for additional information).

1. Provide BVM ventilation or supplemental oxygen as needed.

2. Remember, patients with inadequate breathing **always** get ventilated with the BVM.

B. Manage life-threatening conditions associated with breathing, such as:

1. Flail chest: Provide BVM ventilation.

2. Sucking chest wound: Apply a vented occlusive dressing.

 VII. CIRCULATION

A. Manage obvious life-threatening bleeding immediately.

B. Check pulse, initiate CPR as needed.

C. Check for signs of shock, such as skin condition and capillary refill (in pediatric patients).

 VIII. RAPID SCAN

A. The rapid scan is a quick head-to-toe assessment used specifically to identify any remaining life-threatening conditions not already managed. Examples: signs of internal bleeding, pelvic fracture, femur fracture, traumatic brain injury.

B. The rapid scan should not take longer than 90 seconds. Do **not** be distracted by or focus on non-life-threatening conditions during the rapid scan.

C. The rapid scan should utilize inspection, palpation, and auscultation as needed.

D. The rapid scan includes an assessment of the posterior for life threats.

IX. TRANSPORT PRIORITY

A. Stable or unstable?

1. High transport priority: Unstable patients, including decreased LOC, signs of shock, serious medical condition, severe pain, etc.

2. Stable patients: No obvious life-threatening condition, allowing continued care on the scene prior to transport.

B. Management of high-priority patients

1. Stabilize immediate life threats.

2. Initiate transport to appropriate destination within 10 minutes.

3. Do **not** delay transport of a high-priority patient to manage non-life-threatening conditions.

X. PATIENT HISTORY (see Chapter 8 for detailed information)

A. Identify the chief complaint.

B. Obtain a SAMPLE history.

C. Assess for associated symptoms / pertinent negatives related to the chief complaint, MOI or NOI.

D. *Note:* For conscious medical patients, you will likely begin the patient history right after the primary assessment. For unresponsive patients, high-priority patients, or multi-system trauma patients, you will likely go directly to the secondary assessment/vitals following the primary assessment.

XI. SECONDARY ASSESSMENT

A. The secondary assessment should **not** delay transport of a high-priority patient.

B. The secondary assessment is intended to identify any remaining signs, symptoms, conditions, or injuries not previously discovered and managed.

C. *Note:* All potentially life-threatening conditions should have already been found and managed.

D. Detailed or focused secondary survey

1. The secondary assessment can be a detailed head-to-toe assessment, or it can be a focused exam that assesses only relevant areas.

2. Detailed head-to-toe

   i. Indicated for:

      ➤ Unresponsive patients.

      ➤ Multi-system trauma patients.

      ➤ *Note:* It is not necessary or practical to complete a detailed secondary on every patient.

   ii. Format for detailed secondary

      ➤ Assess head, neck, chest, abdomen, pelvis, extremities, posterior using DCAP-BTLS (**d**eformities, **d**istention, **c**ontusions, **a**brasions, **p**enetrating wounds, **p**aradoxical motion, **b**urns, **t**enderness, **l**acerations, **s**welling).

      ➤ Check all four extremities for pulse, motor response, sensation (PMS).

3. Focused secondary survey

   i. Focuses on only those areas/systems considered relevant to the patient's complaint.

   ii. Indicated for an alert patient with an isolated complaint (trauma or medical).

   iii. The EMT **must** have the knowledge to determine what should be assessed and what can be left out.

4. Baseline vitals

   i. Obtain baseline vitals if not already done.

   ii. Reassess vitals based on patient's condition.

      ➤ Stable patients: every 15 minutes.

      ➤ Unstable patients: every 5 minutes.

XII. REASSESSMENT

A. The reassessment phase is used to continuously monitor the patient's condition for signs of deterioration or improvement.

B. Always begin by reassessing the primary assessment for any changes.

C. Reassess the patient's chief complaint for any changes.

D. Reassess any interventions you performed for signs of improvement or deterioration.

E. Reassess vitals every 5 or 15 minutes depending on the patient's condition.

F. The reassessment phase continues until patient care is transferred, or until it is interrupted because you discover something that requires attention.

XIII. SPECIAL PATIENTS

A. Pediatrics

1. When the situation permits, consider performing a toe-to-head assessment to decrease anxiety.

2. Communicate carefully with pediatric patients. For example, you may tell a child you are going to take his blood pressure, but he may only hear "take your blood."

B. Elderly

1. The history and physical assessment of elderly patients may take more time than normal.

2. Use honorifics (Mr., Mrs., Ms., etc.) unless otherwise directed by the patient.

XIV. SUMMARY OF PATIENT ASSESSMENT

A. Scene size-up

 1. Scene safety

 2. BSI precautions

 3. MOI or NOI

 4. Number of patients

 5. Additional resources

 6. Consider spinal precautions

B. Primary assessment

 1. General impression

 2. LOC

 3. ABC or CAB

 4. Rapid scan as needed

 5. Transport priority

C. Secondary assessment

 1. Detailed head-to-toe or focused exam

 2. Baseline vitals

D. Patient history

 1. SAMPLE history

E. Reassessment

 1. Reassess ABCs

 2. Reassess chief complaint

 3. Reassess interventions

 4. Reassess vitals

PRACTICE QUESTIONS
Answers on page 383.

1. What is the purpose of the primary assessment?

   A. to identify and manage all conditions and injuries prior to transport

   B. to obtain information about the patient's medications and allergies

   C. to identify and manage life-threatening conditions

   D. to reassess the chief complaint, vitals, and interventions

2. You have determined that your patient is unresponsive. You should immediately

   A. check a pulse.

   B. begin compressions.

   C. assess the airway.

   D. transport.

3. What is the purpose of the rapid scan?

   A. to identify all remaining injuries

   B. to determine if CPR is needed

   C. to focus your assessment on areas relevant to the chief complaint

   D. to identify any remaining life-threatening conditions

4. Which of the following are part of the scene size up? (Select the THREE answer options that apply.)

   A. Determine transport priority.

   B. Establish scene safety.

   C. Obtain baseline vitals.

   D. Assess level of consciousness.

   E. Request additional resources.

   F. Identify the MOI or NOI.

5. Which of the following patients should be assessed using the "CAB" approach?

A. Any unresponsive patient.

B. All pediatric patients.

C. Patients responsive to painful stimuli.

D. Trauma patients.

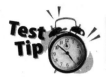

Test Tip

Remember, in addition to the five categories on the national certification exam, you must also stay sharp on patient assessment. Patient assessment will be embedded throughout the test.

Airway, Respiration, and Ventilation

Note: A review of the respiratory section of Chapter 6 is recommended.

I. TERMS TO KNOW

A. **Auscultation:** Listening to sounds from the heart, lungs, or other organs with a stethoscope.

B. **External respiration:** Exchange of oxygen and carbon dioxide between the lungs and the circulatory system.

C. **Hypoxia:** Inadequate delivery of oxygen to the tissues of the body.

D. **Internal respiration:** Exchange of oxygen and carbon dioxide between the circulatory system and the body's cells.

E. **Ventilation:** Movement of air in and out of the lungs.

II. PHYSIOLOGY OF BREATHING

A. Ventilation

1. Ventilation is the movement of air in and out of the lungs; it is observed by chest rise and fall.

2. Normally, ventilation leads to oxygenation, external respiration, and finally, internal respiration.

3. Ventilation is required for oxygenation and respiration; however, it does not ensure them.

4. Inhalation

    i.   This is the active part of ventilation (requires energy).

    ii.   The diaphragm and intercostal muscles contract, intrathoracic pressure decreases (creating negative intrathoracic pressure) and air enters the lungs.

    iii.   Air enters through the upper airway, into the lower airway, and finally into the alveoli.

    iv.   The alveoli are the terminal (final) structure in the lower airway.

    v.   Spontaneous breathing, as described above, is driven by negative pressure, unlike bag-valve-mask ventilation (BVM), which is a form of positive pressure ventilation (PPV).

5. Exhalation

    i.   This is the passive part of ventilation (no energy required).

    ii.   During exhalation, the muscles of respiration relax, the thorax decreases in size, and air is compressed out of the lungs.

6. Regulation of ventilation

    i.   The body's need for oxygen rises and falls based on activity, illness, injury, etc. The brain has two primary methods of controlling oxygen delivery:

        ➤ Rate of ventilation: increasing or decreasing the rate of breathing.

        ➤ Tidal volume: increasing or decreasing the volume of each breath.

    ii. CO_2 drive

        ➤ The carbon dioxide (CO_2) drive is the body's primary system for regulating breathing status.

        ➤ The brain monitors CO_2 levels in the blood and cerebrospinal fluid.

    iii.   Hypoxic drive

        ➤ The hypoxic drive is a backup system to the CO_2 drive.

        ➤ Monitors oxygen levels in plasma.

        ➤ Some patients with chronic obstructive pulmonary disease (COPD) are on the hypoxic drive as they have chronically high levels of CO_2.

> The hypoxic drive can be "fooled" into causing respiratory depression. Patients on the hypoxic drive with prolonged exposure to high concentrations of supplemental oxygen may develop respiratory depression; however, you should **not** withhold oxygen from any severely ill or injured patient.

7. Hypoxia

   i.   Hypoxia is the inadequate delivery of oxygen to the tissues of the body.

   ii. Signs and symptoms of mild (early) hypoxia:

   > Restlessness, anxiety, irritability

   > Dyspnea

   > Tachycardia, tachypnea

   > SpO_2 90% to 94%

   iii. Signs and symptoms of severe (late) hypoxia:

   > Altered or decreased LOC

   > Severe dyspnea

   > Cyanosis

   > Bradycardia (especially in pediatric patients)

   > SpO_2 below 90%

B. Oxygenation

1. Oxygenation is the delivery of oxygen to the blood.

2. Ventilation (spontaneous or assisted) must be adequate for oxygenation to occur.

3. Surrounding air contains about 21% oxygen. Exhaled air contains about 16% oxygen.

4. Administration of supplemental oxygen (nasal cannula, non-rebreather mask, CPAP, etc.) is used to increase the patient's oxygen levels.

5. The nasal cannula (NC), non-rebreather mask (NRB), and continuous positive airway pressure (CPAP) require that the patient have adequate spontaneous ventilation.

C. Respiration

1. Respiration is the exchange of oxygen and carbon dioxide.

2. External respiration: the exchange of oxygen and carbon dioxide between the alveoli and the circulatory system (pulmonary capillaries).

3. Internal respiration: the exchange of oxygen and carbon dioxide between the circulatory system (systemic capillaries) and the body's cells.

III. ASSESSMENT

A. Assessment of breathing includes:

1. *Look:* Look for chest rise and fall.

2. *Listen:* Listen for breathing, ability to speak, auscultate lung sounds.

3. *Feel:* Feel for air movement and chest rise (hand on chest).

B. Adequate breathing

1. Normal respiratory rate and tidal volume

2. Non-labored breathing

3. Clear bilateral lung sounds

C. Inadequate breathing

1. Abnormal rate (too slow or too fast)

2. Shallow chest rise

3. Accessory muscle use

4. Abnormal, diminished, or absent lung sounds

5. Paradoxical motion (flail chest)

6. Dyspnea

7. Accessory muscle use

8. Cyanosis

9. Low SpO_2

10. Agonal breaths (dying gasps) or apnea (no breathing)

D. Auscultation of lung sounds

1. Lung sounds should be assessed on *every* patient. Depending on the situation, lung sounds may be obtained during the primary assessment, during the physical exam, or while assessing vitals.

2. Lung sounds are usually heard better from the patient's back, not the anterior chest.

   i.   Normal: clear lung sounds in both left and right lungs ("clear and equal bilaterally").

   ii. Wheezing: high-pitched whistling sound, typically more noticeable on expiration.

   iii. Crackles/Rales: wet, crackling sounds, usually on inspiration and expiration.

   iv. Rhonchi: low-pitched, congested sounds often due to mucus in the lungs, usually on expiration.

3. Auscultate lung sounds under clothing in three fields:

   i.   Upper lungs (apices): below the clavicles, midclavicular line.

   ii. Middle lung field: middle chest, midclavicular, posterior.

   iii. Lower lungs (base): lower portion of thorax, midclavicular or midaxillary.

   iv. Always auscultate lung sounds from side to side, not top to bottom.

Note: Lung sounds should always be part of your patient assessment. It is especially important with respiratory patients, cardiac patients, trauma patients, and patients with altered mentation or decreased LOC.

E. Pulse oximetry (SpO_2)

1. See Chapter 8 for additional information.

2. Pulse oximetry is part of the standard of care in the prehospital setting.

3. Pulse oximetry should be monitored continuously on significantly ill or injured patients.

4. Treatment goal is to maintain an SpO_2 of at least 95%.

5. The patient's SpO$_2$ should **not** be used to withhold oxygen from a patient in respiratory distress, shock, or other significant illness or injury.

INTERPRETATION SP02

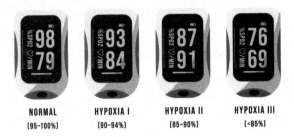

NORMAL	HYPOXIA I	HYPOXIA II	HYPOXIA III
(95-100%)	(90-94%)	(85-90%)	(<85%)

 IV. INTERVENTIONS

A. Airway Management Skills

    1. Remember the order of assessment and management of airway: open the airway, suction the airway, secure the airway ("open-suction-secure").

    2. Manually open the airway (as needed).

        i. Head-tilt, chin-lift (no spinal injury suspected)

        ii. Jaw thrust maneuvers (suspected spinal cord injury)

B. Suction

    1. Suction the upper airway as needed

        i. Aspiration (entry of matter in the lungs) can cause aspiration pneumonia. About 1 in 5 patients with aspiration pneumonia will die.

        ii. Suction is indicated if there are secretions (blood, vomit, mucus, etc.) in the airway that could be aspirated, obstruct the airway, interfere with ventilations or insertion of an airway adjunct.

        iii. Larger substances that cannot be suctioned (debris, foreign body, teeth, food, etc.) should be removed manually.

        iv. Suction is performed, when indicated, after manually opening the airway and before insertion of an airway adjunct.

2. Suction units

    i.   All suction units should have a disposable canister.

    ii.   Suction units should be able to generate a vacuum of 300 mmHg when tubing is clamped.

3. Suction catheters

    i.   A suction catheter attaches to the suction unit and is inserted into the patient's airway.

    ii.   Suction catheters, tubing, and canister should all be single-patient use (disposable).

    iii.   Rigid suction catheters are also called "tonsil tip" or "Yankauer." These are designed to suction the oral airway.

    iv.   French catheters are flexible and come in several sizes. These are designed to suction the nose, stoma, or the inside of an advanced airway.

4. Suction procedures

    i.   Suctioning increases the risk of hypoxia and delays subsequent interventions, so time is limited. Do not suction longer than . . .

       ➤ Adults: Do not exceed 15 seconds.

       ➤ Children: Do not exceed 10 seconds.

       ➤ Infants: Do not exceed 5 seconds.

    ii.   Insert rigid (Yankauer) catheter only as far as you can see.

    iii.   Measure French suction catheter depth by measuring from corner of the mouth to the earlobe.

    iv.   Apply suction as you withdraw the catheter (not as you insert catheter).

    v.   Run sterile water through suction catheter and tubing after use to prevent blockage.

C. Mechanical airway adjunct (as needed)

1. Oropharyngeal airway (OPA)

    i.   OPAs are **only** for unresponsive patients. Inserting an OPA in responsive patients can stimulate the gag reflex, cause vomiting, and aspiration.

ii. OPAs are intended to prevent the tongue from obstructing the upper airway in supine, unresponsive patients.

iii. Measure OPA prior to insertion. Measure from corner of mouth to earlobe.

iv. Adult OPA insertion: Manually open airway first, suction as needed, then insert upside down with distal end pointing toward roof of mouth. Rotate 180 degrees and advance into place. Flange (flat part) should rest on patient's lips.

v. Pediatric OPA insertion: Manually open airway first, suction as needed. Depress tongue with a tongue depressor and insert directly into place (no rotation). Alternate technique: Insert OPA sideways and rotate 90 degrees into place.

vi. Immediately remove OPA if patient begins to gag. Have suction ready.

2. Nasopharyngeal airway (NPA)

i. NPAs can be used in patients who are not unconscious (an advantage over OPAs). NPAs work well in patients who are responsive to pain, with intact gag reflex, but still at risk of airway obstruction from the tongue.

ii. Contraindications for NPA (do **not** use):

➤ Do not insert an NPA in patients who are awake and capable of protecting their own airway.

➤ Do not insert an NPA in patients with severe head injury or facial trauma.

➤ Do not force the NPA when you meet resistance to insertion (try other nostril).

iii. Sizing NPA: Measure from tip of nose to earlobe. *Note:* NPAs are not typically used in patients under about one year of age.

iv. Inserting the NPA

➤ Lubricate with water-soluble lubricant **only**. Never use petroleum-based products.

➤ Always insert with bevel (angled end) toward the septum.

➤ Try larger nostril first. Switch if resistance is felt.

➤ Advance gently, rotating as necessary. Do **not** force.

➤ Remove immediately if patient begins to gag. Have suction ready.

Note: While many EMS systems allow EMTs to utilize supraglottic airway devices (such as the i-gel), it is not currently part of the National EMS Scope of Practice for EMTs. For more information, see *www.ems.gov/assets/National_ EMS_Scope_of_Practice_Model_2019.pdf.*

   D. Supplemental oxygen

     1. The goal of supplemental oxygen administration is to maintain an SpO_2 above 94%.

     2. Oxygen is typically not indicated if the patient is alert, stable, has no respiratory distress or signs of shock, and has an SpO_2 of 95% or greater.

Note: A low SpO_2 reading may be reason enough to administer supplemental oxygen; however, a normal SpO_2 reading alone is **not** a reason to withhold oxygen from patients who show other signs of hypoxia, shock, etc.

     3. Indications for supplemental oxygen

       i. All patients in cardiac or respiratory arrest

       ii. All patients receiving BVM ventilation

       iii. All patients with suspected hypoxia (dyspnea, cyanosis, etc.)

       iv. All patients with signs of shock

       v. All patients with an SpO_2 of less than 95%

       vi. All patients with an altered or decreased LOC

       vii. If in doubt, it is better to administer oxygen than to withhold it. Follow local protocol.

     4. Do **not** administer oxygen if the environment is unsafe, such as near an open flame.

Note: American Heart Association guidelines recommend that patients with suspected acute coronary syndrome or stroke **not** receive oxygen unless they have an SpO_2 of less than 94%, or complain of dyspnea, or have signs of shock or heart failure. If a pulse oximeter is not available, oxygen should be administered.

5. Oxygen cylinders (tanks)

   i.   Oxygen cylinders are seamless, aluminum, green, and come in various sizes.

   ii. Oxygen tanks should never be left standing unattended.

   iii. Oxygen cylinders and flow meters (regulators) use a pin indexing system to prevent non-oxygen regulators from accidentally being connected to an oxygen cylinder.

   iv. The amount of oxygen in a cylinder is measured in pounds per square inch (psi).

   ➤ A full tank is 2,000 psi.

   ➤ Replace or refill the tank at 200 psi (this is known as the safe residual pressure).

6. Flow meters (regulators)

   i.   Flow meters are connected to the oxygen cylinder and reduce the pressure coming from the tank to safe levels. The regulator allows the selection of a specific flow rate, measured in liters per minute (L/min or lpm).

7. Nonrebreather (NRB) mask

   i.   Referred to as "high-flow" oxygen.

   ii. NRB masks come in adult and pediatric sizes.

   iii. NRB masks are typically set to at least 10 lpm (as needed to keep reservoir filled with oxygen).

   iv. Patients on a NRB mask receive about 90% oxygen.

   v.   Cautions:

   ➤ The reservoir must be full before applying the mask.

   ➤ Never administer less than 10 lpm.

   ➤ If the reservoir completely deflates during inhalation, the flow rate should be increased.

   ➤ Immediately remove the mask if oxygen source is lost.

   ➤ NRB mask is for patients who are breathing adequately but require supplemental oxygen.

8. Nasal cannula (NC)

   i.   Referred to as "low-flow" oxygen.

    ii. Indicated for patients who are breathing adequately but require supplemental oxygen (and high-flow oxygen isn't necessary or isn't tolerated).

    iii. Patients who feel claustrophobic from NRB mask may better tolerate a nasal cannula.

    iv. Flow rate: 1 to 6 lpm.

    v. Patients on a nasal cannula receive about 24% to 45% oxygen, depending on the lpm delivered. Each liter of oxygen by nasal cannula increases the 21% oxygen in atmospheric air by 3% to 4%. Example:

      ➤ 1 lpm by NC = about 24%–25% oxygen

      ➤ 2 lpm by NC = about 27%–29% oxygen

      ➤ 3 lpm by NC = about 30%–33% oxygen

      ➤ 4 lpm by NC = about 33%–37% oxygen

      ➤ 5 lpm by NC = about 36%–41% oxygen

      ➤ 6 lpm by NC = about 39%–45% oxygen

    vi. *Caution:* Prolonged use can dry out and irritate nasal passages if oxygen is not humidified.

9. Venturi mask

    i. Venturi masks deliver specific concentrations of low-flow oxygen.

    ii. Not commonly used in EMS.

10. High-flow nasal oxygen (HFNO)

    i. HFNO is an emerging therapy that delivers CPAP-like support to reduce the patient's work of breathing.

    ii. HFNO is simple to use and well-tolerated; however, it requires a tremendous amount of oxygen (40–70 lpm).

11. Hazards of oxygen administration

    i. Oxygen is combustible. **Never** use oxygen near an open flame, cigarettes, etc.

    ii. Oxygen tanks are highly pressurized and must be handled cautiously. **Never** leave an oxygen tank standing unattended.

    iii. Supplemental oxygen administration in suspected myocardial infarction or stroke patients who were **not** hypoxic does not appear to reduce mortality.

    iv. Long-term exposure to high concentrations of oxygen in newborns can cause retinal damage.

    v. Respiratory depression is a risk for COPD patients who are on the hypoxic drive; however, it typically requires long-term exposure to high-concentration oxygen. Do **not** withhold oxygen from any hypoxic patient.

E. Assisted Ventilation

1. Also called positive pressure ventilation (PPV) or artificial ventilation. Includes:

    i. Mouth-to-mask (pocket mask) ventilation

    ii. Bag-valve-mask (BVM) ventilation

2. Indications:

    i. Any patient with inadequate spontaneous breathing

    ii. Patients breathing less than 10 times per minute or over 30 times per minute

    iii. Cardiac arrest (no pulse, no breathing)

    iv. Respiratory arrest (no breathing)

    v. Agonal breathing (dying gasps)

    vi. Severe respiratory distress, respiratory failure (inadequate spontaneous breathing)

    vii. Severe bradypnea (slow breathing) or severe tachypnea (rapid breathing)

3. Remember, airway always comes before breathing. The airway should be assessed and appropriately managed before initiating PPV.

4. Complications of PPV

    i. Hyperventilation is a common and dangerous complication of PPV, especially with a BVM device.

        ➤ Occurs when rescuers ventilate too fast, too forcefully, or both.

> ➤ Hyperventilation leads to gastric distention (excessive air in the stomach), vomiting, and aspiration. Aspiration pneumonia significantly increases the risk of death.

> ➤ Hyperventilation also appears to significantly increase intrathoracic pressure and decrease coronary perfusion, which decrease survival rates for cardiac arrest patients.

> ➤ Research indicates that **most** rescuers excessively ventilate patients during out-of-hospital cardiac arrest.

5. Pocket mask barrier device

   i.   A pocket mask barrier device is a mask placed between the patient and the provider during artificial ventilations.

   ii. Advantages: Most pocket masks are small and easy to use (much easier than a BVM).

   iii. Disadvantages: There is a greater biohazard exposure risk than with a BVM, and it only delivers 16% oxygen (unless connected to oxygen source).

6. BVM ventilation

   i.   BVM ventilation is the primary means of providing PPV to patients in the prehospital setting.

   ii. Advantages of BVM

   > ➤ When used correctly and connected to oxygen, the patient receives over 90% oxygen.

   > ➤ Reduced biohazard exposure risk compared to mouth-to-mask.

   > ➤ Self-inflating BVMs do not require an oxygen source to function.

   > ➤ Can be used with a mask or an advanced airway device.

   iii. Disadvantages

   > ➤ Effective single-rescuer operation (while avoiding hyperventilation) requires a high degree of proficiency.

   > ➤ Rescuers are highly prone to hyperventilating patients with the BVM.

Note: A National Institutes of Health (NIH) study found that over 90% of healthcare providers unintentionally hyperventilated patients when using the BVM device.

iv. Sizes and volumes of BVM devices

➤ Infant BVM: 150–280 mL

➤ Child BVM: 500–700 mL

➤ Adult BVM: 1,000–1,600 mL

➤ *Note:* There are at least six different mask sizes for the BVM device, from newborn to adult.

v. Components of BVM

➤ Self-inflating bag

➤ Clear masks of various sizes

➤ Oxygen reservoir and tubing

➤ The entire BVM should be single patient use (disposable)

➤ *Note:* Most pediatric BVM devices have a pressure relief ("pop-off") valve. They are meant to avoid over-pressurization during ventilation; however, they can prevent adequate ventilation. Follow local protocols regarding use/disabling of pop-off valves.

vi. Correct tidal volume

➤ Gentle rise and fall of the chest during PPV is the best way to assess adequate ventilation.

➤ It should take about one second to inflate the chest with the BVM. Squeezing the bag too fast increases the risk of gastric distention.

➤ BVM ventilations are typically performed much better with two rescuers: one rescuer with two hands on the bag, and one rescuer with two hands on the mask.

vii. Correct rates of ventilation for apneic patients with a pulse

➤ Adults (with or without advanced airway): one breath every six seconds (10 breaths/minute)

➤ Infants and children (with or without advanced airway): one breath every two to three seconds (20 to 30 breaths/minute)

➤ Newborns: 40 to 60 breaths per minute

viii. Patients in cardiac arrest (compression to ventilation ratios)

➤ Adults (one- or two-rescuer CPR): 30 compressions and 2 breaths (30:2)

> ➤ Single-rescuer CPR (children & infants): 30 compressions and 2 breaths (30:2)

> ➤ Two-rescuer CPR (infants, children): 15 compressions and 2 breaths (15:2)

> ➤ Newborns: 3 compressions and 1 breath (3:1)

> ➤ *Note:* It is not necessary to pause compressions for ventilations once an advanced airway has been placed.

Note: If you are not sure whether your patient needs BVM ventilation or not, then do it. If you're wrong, the patient will find a way to let you know. If you fail to ventilate a patient who needs it, the patient will continue to deteriorate.

F. Continuous Positive Airway Pressure (CPAP)

1. CPAP is a form of non-invasive ventilation.

2. CPAP is used to treat patients in significant respiratory distress due to congestive heart failure or reactive airway disease.

3. Provides air pressure to patient during inhalation and exhalation. This can ease breathing and help keep the bronchioles and alveoli open. CPAP helps relieve pulmonary edema (fluid in the lungs).

4. Requires a pressure-tight mask over the patient's mouth and nose.

5. Many patients feel relief almost immediately.

6. There are several contraindications for CPAP, such as hypotension, vomiting, and apnea.

7. CPAP is **not** a substitute for BVM ventilation; however, CPAP may help patients avoid needing BVM ventilation.

8. Patients **must** be breathing spontaneously and able to follow commands.

9. Follow local protocol regarding use of CPAP.

G. Bilevel Positive Airway Pressure (BiPAP)

1. BiPAP is similar to CPAP; however, it provides two levels of non-invasive pressure (one during inhalation and one during exhalation).

2. BiPAP is highly effective at reducing the patient's work of breathing.

V. SPECIAL PATIENT SITUATIONS

A. Follow local protocol regarding use of automated transport ventilators.

B. Routine suctioning of neonates at birth is **not** recommended. It can cause bradycardia and apnea.

C. Infants and children

    1. Anatomical and physiological differences from adults

        i. The pediatric airway is more easily obstructed (the tongue is larger in proportion to the airway).

        ii. The pediatric head is larger in proportion to the body. Pad behind the supine pediatric patient's shoulders to maintain airway alignment.

        iii. The lungs are smaller. Take great care to avoid hyperventilation.

        iv. Hypoxia can develop rapidly in pediatric patients. They have less oxygen reserves and higher metabolic rates.

        v. Place infants and toddlers in the "sniffing" position (without hyperextension of the neck) during positive pressure ventilation.

        vi. Infants and younger children may require padding under the shoulders to prevent hyperflexion of the neck while supine.

Note: Beware of bradycardia in pediatric patients! Bradycardia in pediatric patients is a sign of hypoxia until proven otherwise.

    2. Hypoxia and respiratory failure in pediatric patients

        i. Pediatric patients are often resistant to having an oxygen mask on their face. Consider "blow-by" oxygen (holding the mask or oxygen tubing close to the patient's face).

        ii. Bradycardia is common in pediatric patients experiencing significant hypoxia. Always assess any pediatric patient with bradycardia for hypoxia.

        iii. Airway or respiratory problems and shock are the primary causes of circulatory collapse in pediatric patients.

        iv. Ominous signs of respiratory failure in pediatric patients

            ➤ Bradycardia and poor muscle tone

> ➤ Decreased LOC

> ➤ Head bobbing

> ➤ Grunting on exhalation

> ➤ "Seesaw" breathing

    v. Place infants and toddlers who need BVM ventilation in a "sniffing" position without hyperextension of the neck.

D. Patients with tracheostomy tube or stoma

  1. A tracheal stoma is a surgical opening in the neck into the trachea.

  2. A tracheostomy tube ("trach tube") is a curved tube inserted into a tracheal stoma directly into the trachea.

  3. Patients with a tracheal stoma (with or without a trach tube) who need supplemental oxygen should have an oxygen mask placed over the stoma (not the face).

  4. To ventilate a patient with a tracheal stoma (and no trach tube), use an infant or pediatric mask (allows for seal around the stoma) and the appropriate size BVM device.

  5. To ventilate a patient with a trach tube, remove the mask from the BVM and connect the BVM directly to the trach tube.

  6. Trach tubes and stomas can become easily obstructed with mucus. Have suction (French catheter) ready.

E. Foreign body airway obstruction (FBAO)

  1. Remember, the tongue is the leading cause of airway obstruction; however, vomit, food, toys, etc., can also obstruct the airway.

  2. Indications of complete or nearly complete FBAO

    i. Inability to cough, speak, or breathe

    ii. Clutching the throat (conscious patients)

    iii. Inability to ventilate the patient despite repositioning airway and managing the tongue (unconscious patients)

  3. Management of FBAO

    i. Conscious adults and children: Perform abdominal thrusts until the obstruction is relieved or until the patient loses consciousness.

ii. Conscious infant: Alternate between five back slaps and five chest thrusts until the obstruction is relieved or the patient loses consciousness.

iii. Unconscious (all ages): Perform chest compressions. Before attempting ventilations, inspect the airway for visible foreign bodies. Remove them if you're able.

F. Dentures

1. Dentures are usually secured in place and can be left alone.

2. If loose, they should be removed.

3. *Note:* It is much easier to ventilate a patient with dentures in place.

PRACTICE QUESTIONS
Answers on page 384.

1. You have just initiated BVM ventilations for your apneic patient. Which of the following would **best** help determine if the patient is being ventilated effectively? (Select the THREE answer options that apply.)

A. Check pupillary response.

B. Assess for chest rise and fall.

C. Monitor SpO_2.

D. Auscultate lung sounds.

E. Assess distal pulses.

F. Assess BP.

2. Your 9-month-old patient is lethargic and has a pulse of 62 beats per minute. You should suspect that the baby is

A. sleeping.

B. hypoxic.

C. in cardiac arrest.

D. mildly dehydrated.

3. Which of the following indicates the need for supplemental oxygen by nasal cannula or nonrebreather mask?

   A. warm, dry skin

   B. agonal breathing

   C. an SpO_2 of 92%

   D. clear, bilateral lung sounds

4. Your patient is responsive only to painful stimuli. The airway is clear. You should first

   A. insert an NPA.

   B. insert an OPA.

   C. suction the airway.

   D. begin BVM ventilations.

5. Your patient has a tracheostomy tube and is showing signs of hypoxia. To administer supplemental oxygen, you should

   A. remove the trach tube.

   B. place a NRB on the patient's face.

   C. apply a nasal cannula at 6 lpm.

   D. place an oxygen mask over the trach tube.

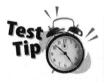

Test Tip

The certification exam will include many scenario-based questions. These can be mentally draining. Read each question carefully. Look for key information. There is usually something specific in the question that will point you to the correct answer. Read all the answer choices before making your selection.

PART IV

PHARMACOLOGY, CARDIOLOGY, AND RESUSCITATION/STROKE

REVIEW PLUS
END-OF-CHAPTER PRACTICE

Pharmacology

I. TERMS TO KNOW

A. Adrenergic: Refers to the sympathetic nervous system.

B. Agonist: Medications that stimulate an effect.

C. Antagonist: Medications that inhibit an effect.

D. Drug profile: Provides the essential information about a drug.

E. Cholinergic: Refers to the parasympathetic nervous system.

II. PHARMACOKINETICS AND PHARMACODYNAMICS

A. Pharmacokinetics is the study of how drugs enter the body, and how they are metabolized and eliminated.

B. Pharmacodynamics is the study of a drug's effects on the body.

III. THE "DRUG PROFILE"

A. The drug profile provides the essential information about a drug.

1. Drug name: Trade name(s) and generic name.

2. Drug class: The "family" the drug belongs to, such as vasodilator, bronchodilator, pain reliever, etc.

3. Mechanism of action (MOA): Describes how the drug does what it does. For example, nitroglycerine dilates blood vessels, oral glucose raises blood glucose levels, etc.

I. Agonists: medications that stimulate an effect, such as a bronchodilator medication in an inhaler.

ii. Sympathomimetics (also called adrenergic drugs) mimic effects of the sympathetic nervous system (fight-or-flight). Example: epinephrine (adrenalin) is an adrenergic drug that has three distinct agonist effects:

> ➤ Alpha 1 agonists increase peripheral vascular resistance by stimulating peripheral vasoconstriction. This helps increase blood pressure in patients experiencing anaphylaxis.

> ➤ Beta 1 agonists increase heart rate and cardiac force of contraction. This helps increase cardiac output and BP in patients experiencing anaphylaxis.

> ➤ Beta 2 agonists stimulate bronchodilation. This can improve ventilation and oxygenation in patients experiencing anaphylaxis.

iii. Antagonists: Medications that inhibit an effect.

> ➤ Anticholinergic medications inhibit effects of the parasympathetic nervous system. Example: Atropine can reverse the effects of cholinergic (parasympathetic nervous system) poisoning. This can be lifesaving when exposed to a nerve agent or organophosphate pesticides.

> ➤ Naloxone is also an antagonist medication that reverses the effects of an opioid overdose.

4. Indications: Situations where the drug should be considered for administration, such as oxygen for a patient who is hypoxic, or nitroglycerine for a patient with chest pain.

5. Contraindications: Situations where the drug should not be given, even if it is indicated.

i. Example: Nitroglycerine cannot be given to a patient who is hypotensive, even if the patient is experiencing chest pain.

ii. Some drugs have "relative" contraindications that allow for some discretion. Typically, this applies to situations where withholding the drug may be more harmful than administering it.

6. Route of administration and dose

   i. Route of administration: This is how the drug is administered, such as oral, sublingual, intranasal, intramuscular, etc.

     ➤ Enteral: Enteral drugs enter the body through the digestive system (oral medications).

     ➤ Parenteral: Parenteral drugs enter the body through any means other than enteral (sublingual, inhaled, intramuscular, etc.).

   ii. Dose: The amount of drug that should be given (Example: 6 lpm by nasal cannula, or 0.4 mg of nitroglycerine sublingual).

7. Side effects: These are any effects the drug may have other than the desired/intended effects.

   i. Example: Headache is a known side effect of nitroglycerine.

   ii. Untoward effects: Untoward effects are potentially dangerous side effects, such as hypotension following nitroglycerine administration.

8. Supply: This is the form and concentration in which the drug is carried by the EMT. For example, oral glucose: 15 gram tube; nitroglycerine: 0.4 mg tablets; epinephrine: 0.3 mg auto-injector.

9. Special considerations: any information unique to a specific drug that providers should be aware of. For example, nitroglycerine is heat and light sensitive and should be stored in a cool, dry place out of direct sunlight.

B. EMTs should know the locally approved drug profile for all medications they are allowed to administer.

IV. ONSET, PEAK, DURATION OF ACTION

A. Onset: How long it takes a medication to begin having the desired effect.

B. Peak: How long until the medication reaches its peak effects.

C. Duration: How long a medication will maintain the desired effect.

V. ROUTES OF ADMINISTRATION

A. Enteral: oral (PO)

1. Slow onset of action

2. Safe, but unpredictable absorption

3. Examples: aspirin, oral glucose

B. Parenteral routes (used by EMTs)

1. Intramuscular (IM)

   i. Injection directly into the muscle.

   ii. Rapid absorption—faster than oral, but not as fast as intravenous (IV) or intraosseous (IO). IV and IO routes are used by advanced-level providers.

   iii. Examples: epinephrine auto-injector, atropine auto-injector, DuoDote auto-injector, naloxone auto-injector.

2. Inhalation

   i. Inhaled into the lungs

   ii. Rapid onset

   iii. Examples: oxygen, inhaler medications such as albuterol

3. Intranasal (IN)

   i. Through the nose

   ii. Rapid onset of action. Often administered using a mucosal atomizer device (MAD).

   iii. Examples: naloxone. Additional IN medications for EMT use are likely coming.

4. Sublingual (SL)

   i. Under the tongue

   ii. Faster onset than oral. *Note:* Sublingual medications are rapidly absorbed by the tissue under the tongue. Sublingual medications bypass the digestive system; however, they are given by mouth. As a result, SL may be considered either enteral or parenteral.

   iii. Example: nitroglycerine.

VI. MEDICATION FORMS

A. Tablets or capsules: pill forms typically administered orally (PO), such as aspirin, nitroglycerine, acetaminophen, etc.

B. Solutions: medications in liquid form, such as epinephrine, nitroglycerine, naloxone, atropine.

C. Metered dose inhaler (MDI) or small-volume nebulizer (SVN): medications that are aerosolized and inhaled.

D. Gels: semiliquid medications, such as oral glucose

E. Gas: medications in gas form, such as oxygen

VII. ADMINISTERING MEDICATIONS

A. EMTs must have written protocols or online medical direction allowing them to administer medications.

B. Be sure the medication you are preparing to administer is not expired, damaged, or contaminated.

C. History and physical

1. In most cases, it is important to obtain a thorough patient history, vitals, and complete a physical exam prior to administering medications.

2. Determine what medications the patient takes regularly or has taken to treat the current complaint.

3. Determine if the patient has any allergies to medications.

D. The Six Rights of medication administration

1. Right patient: Be sure the drug is administered to the right patient.

2. Right drug: Be sure the patient receives the correct medication.

3. Right route: Be sure the drug is administered properly.

4. Right amount: Be sure the patient receives the correct dose.

5. Right time: Be sure the patient receives the medication at the correct time.

6. Right documentation: Thoroughly document all relevant information about the medication administration, including the patient's response to the medication.

E. It is highly recommended that you consult with another EMS provider on scene to ensure that the Six Rights are being followed.

Note: It is critical that you know specifically what you want a medication to make happen or stop from happening before you administer it. After administration, you must reassess the patient to see whether the desired effect was achieved, or whether the patient experienced any side effects. Document thoroughly!

 ## VIII. REASSESSMENT

A. Determine whether the medication had the desired effect.

B. Determine whether the patient experienced any side effects from the medication.

C. Document!

 ## IX. MEDICATIONS ADMINISTERED BY EMTs

A. The medications that an EMT can administer are determined by local protocol, the state EMS authority, and medical direction. This varies widely across jurisdictions.

B. **Always** follow local protocols and consult medical direction with any questions or concerns.

C. Medications typically administered by EMTs:

1. activated charcoal (**not** used by EMTs in many jurisdictions)

2. aspirin

3. atropine (auto-injector)

4. bronchodilators such as albuterol (MDI)

5. epinephrine (auto-injector)

6. naloxone (auto-injector or intranasal)

7. nitroglycerine (typically not carried by EMT; must be prescribed to patient)

8. oral glucose

9. over-the-counter analgesics, such as acetaminophen

10. oxygen

 ## X. SPECIAL PATIENTS

A. Pediatric patients

1. Medication dosages for pediatric patients are often weight-based.

2. About 20% of pediatric patients who receive activated charcoal will vomit, increasing the risk of aspiration and dehydration.

B. Elderly patients

1. The potency of some medications is increased in elderly patients.

2. It often takes longer to process medications through the body for elimination. This increases the risk of overdose.

3. Many elderly patients are on four or more prescription medications, increasing the risk of drug interaction.

XI. DRUG PROFILES

Note: The following drug profiles provide general information about the medications. Most states have drug profiles that are approved by the state EMS authority. **Always** follow your protocols.

Drug Profiles

Name(s)	Class	MOA	Indications
Activated charcoal • Actidose • CharcoalAid • Liqui-Char • Super-Char	Adsorbent	Adheres (binds) many drugs and chemicals, reducing absorption from the GI tract	Recently ingested poisons
Aspirin • ASA • Anacin • Bayer	• Anti-inflammatory • Anti-platelet aggregate • Antipyretic	• Reduces inflammation • Reduces clot formation • Reduces fever	Chest pain
Atropine • Rafa auto-injector	Anticholinergic	Blocks para-sympathetic nervous system	Poisoning due to nerve agent or organo-phosphates in patients at least 6 months old
MDI broncho-dilators • Albuterol • Proventil • Ventolin	Bronchodilators	Relaxes bronchial smooth muscle	Dyspnea due to asthma, reactive airway disease
Epinephrine autoinjector • EpiPen • Auvi-Q	• Sympatho-mimetic • Broncho-dilator	• Peripheral vaso-constriction • Increased heart rate • Broncho-dilation	Anaphylaxis
Naloxone • Narcan • Evzio	Opioid antagonist	Reverses effects of opioids/narcotics	Suspected opioid overdose
Nitroglycerine • Nitrostat • Nitrolingual • NitroMist	• Anti-anginal • Vasodilator	Vasodilation	Chest pain
Oral glucose • Glucose • Insta-Glucose	Oral hyperglycemic	Increases blood glucose levels	Hypoglycemia
OTC analgesics	Follow local protocol	Follow local protocol	Follow local protocol
Oxygen	See Chapter 10	See Chapter 10	See Chapter 10

Drug Profiles (cont'd)

Contra-indications	Dose and Route	Side Effects	Supply
• Decreased LOC • Inability to swallow • Ingestion of acids, alkalis, or hydrocarbons	25–50 grams PO	• Nausea & vomiting	15, 25, 50 gram bottles or tubes
• Decreased LOC • Inability to swallow • Bleeding, ulcer • Pediatric patients	162–324 mg PO (2–4 chewables of 81 mg each)	• Usually none in adults • Stomach pain • Increased bleeding Allergic reaction • Do **NOT** administer to pediatrics	81 mg chewable tablets
Infants under 6 months (15 lbs.)	**Age 6 months to 4 years:** • 0.5 mg IM **Age 5 to 10 years:** • 1 mg IM **Over age 10:** • 2 mg IM	• Tachycardia • Dry mouth • Blurred vision • Headache • Palpitations	0.5 mg, 1 mg, 2 mg auto-injector
• Unable to follow commands • Respiratory failure	One to two inhalations from MDI	Tachycardia Hyper-tension Anxiety	MDI
None	**Adult:** 0.3 mg auto-injector IM **Peds (under 66 lbs):** 0.15 mg peds auto-injector IM	• Tachy-cardia • Hyper-tension • Anxiety	**Adult:** 0.3 mg auto-injector **Peds:** 0.15 mg auto-injector
None	**IN:** 4 mg **IM:** 0.4–2 mg auto-injector	• Combative • Withdrawal symptoms	Nasal spray and IM auto injector
• Not prescribed to patient • Hypotension • Use of medications for erectile dysfunction • Head injury • Pediatrics	0.4 mg SL tablet or spray	• Tachycardia • Hypo-tension • Headache • Burning under tongue	Tablets or spray (0.4 mg each)
• Decreased LOC • Unable to swallow	Half to one tube PO	Aspiration risk	15–45 gram tubes
• Follow local protocol	Follow local protocol	Follow local protocol	Follow local protocol
See Chapter 10	See Chapter 10	See Chapter 10	See Chapter 10

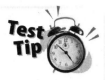

PRACTICE QUESTIONS
Answers on page 385.

1. Which of the following medications are administered parenterally? (Select the THREE answer options that apply.)

   A. aspirin

   B. epinephrine

   C. acetaminophen (Tylenol)

   D. atropine

   E. oral glucose

   F. oxygen

2. Which of the following medications is used to reverse the effects of an opioid overdose?

   A. naloxone

   B. atropine

   C. albuterol

   D. nitroglycerine

3. Which of the following side effects of nitroglycerine is of greatest concern?

   A. headache

   B. burning under the tongue

   C. hypotension

   D. relief of chest pain

4. EMTs typically do NOT carry which of the following medications?

   A. oxygen

   B. oral glucose

   C. naloxone

   D. nitroglycerine

5. Which of the following medications may be used for recently ingested poisons?

   A. activated charcoal

   B. aspirin

   C. oral glucose

   D. nitroglycerine

Cardiac Emergencies and Resuscitation

Note: A review of the circulatory section of Chapter 6 is recommended.

I. TERMS TO KNOW

A. **Acute coronary syndrome:** Conditions caused by acute reduction of blood flow to the heart.

B. **Angina:** Transient chest pain due to lack of oxygen to the heart muscle.

C. **Diaphoresis:** Excessive sweating.

D. **Myocardial infarction:** A heart attack.

E. **Silent heart attack:** A heart attack where the patient doesn't complain of chest pain.

II. PATHOPHYSIOLOGY

A. Heart attack is the leading cause of death in the United States.

B. Rapid, effective initiation of CPR can double survival rates from out-of-hospital cardiac arrest.

III. CARDIAC EMERGENCIES

A. Acute Coronary Syndrome (ACS)

   1. ACS is any condition caused by acute reduction in blood flow to the heart, including:

      i. Acute myocardial infarction (AMI): This is a heart attack.

      ii. Unstable angina: unpredictable onset and unrelieved by rest.

   2. Most (but not all) patients with ACS will have chest pain.

B. Angina

   1. Angina (aka angina pectoris) is transient chest pain caused by a lack of oxygen to the heart muscle (myocardium).

   2. The heart's demand for oxygen temporarily exceeds the supply due to inadequate blood flow through the coronary arteries (myocardial ischemia).

   3. Typically caused by plaque buildup in coronary arteries (atherosclerosis).

   4. Signs and symptoms

      i. Chest pain, usually during physical activity or stress.

      ii. Pain usually resolves with rest or nitroglycerine and usually lasts less than 10 minutes (unless patient experiencing unstable angina).

      iii. Does not cause permanent damage (unlike myocardial infarction); however, it should be treated as a serious cardiac condition.

   5. Unstable angina

      i. A less common, and more serious, form of angina.

      ii. Unpredictable onset (not exercise or stress induced) and unrelieved by rest.

      iii. Signs and symptoms are very similar to myocardial infarction.

      iv. Treat as a cardiac emergency.

C. Acute Myocardial Infarction (AMI or MI)

   1. Heart disease is the leading cause of death in the U.S. (about 700,000 deaths per year).

2. A myocardial infarction (heart attack) is death to an area of the myocardium (heart muscle) due to lack of oxygenated blood flow through the coronary arteries.

3. Dead heart muscle becomes scar tissue and can no longer contribute to cardiac contraction.

4. The time from the onset of cardiac damage to restoration of blood flow through the coronary arteries is critical to minimizing the size of the infarction (dead heart muscle).

5. Signs and symptoms of MI

    i.   Chest pain

    ii.   Weakness

    iii. Dyspnea

    iv.   Diaphoresis (excessive sweating)

    v.   Pallor (pale)

    vi.   Feeling of impending doom or denial

    vii. Abnormal vitals

    viii. Sudden cardiac arrest

6. Angina vs. MI

    i.   Always treat for the possibility of MI.

    ii.   MI pain does not go away on its own. Angina pain often resolves in about 10 minutes with rest or nitroglycerine.

    iii. MI pain and unstable angina pain can occur at any time. Regular angina typically occurs during times of exertion or stress.

7. Atypical MI presentations

    i.   Not all patients experiencing an MI have chest pain.

        ➤ An MI without pain is called a "silent MI."

        ➤ Silent MI patients often complain of weakness, epigastric pain, or indigestion.

    ii.   Patient populations that are more likely to present with atypical MI:

        ➤ Elderly patients

        ➤ Women

➤ Diabetics

➤ Alcoholics

8. Complications of MI

   i. Cardiac dysrhythmias (irregular heartbeat)

   ii. Sudden cardiac arrest

   iii. Congestive heart failure (CHF) due to decreased pumping efficiency of the heart

   iv. Cardiogenic shock (pump failure)

D. Congestive Heart Failure

1. CHF occurs when the heart is no longer able to pump effectively. This causes fluid to back up in the cardiovascular system.

   i. Left heart failure

     ➤ The left ventricle can no longer pump effectively.

     ➤ Fluid backs up to the lungs (pulmonary capillaries).

     ➤ Left heart failure often leads to right heart failure.

     ➤ Signs and symptoms

       — Pulmonary edema (wet lung sounds aka rales)

       — Dyspnea, especially on exertion, at night, or while supine

       — Cough

   ii. Right heart failure

     ➤ The right ventricle can no longer pump effectively.

     ➤ Fluid backs up into the venous system.

     ➤ Left heart failure is a common cause of right heart failure.

     ➤ Signs and symptoms

       — Jugular venous distension (JVD when seated

       — Pedal edema (foot and ankle swelling)

Note: Remember, JVD is common in supine patients. JVD in seated patients may be an indication of various medical problems, such as right heart failure, cardiac tamponade, tension pneumothorax, or pulmonary embolism. **Always** assess lung sounds for any patient with abnormal JVD.

   E. Hypertension

      1. Review Chapter 8 for details regarding normal BP, elevated BP, and stage 1 and stage 2 hypertension.

      2. Always assess patients with an abnormal BP for associated signs and symptoms, such as:

         i.   Headache

         ii. Blurred vision

         iii. Nausea

         iv. Nosebleed

         v. Dizziness or syncope

         vi. Tinnitus (ringing in the ears)

         vii. Hypertensive crisis

            ➤ Systolic BP higher than 180 and/or diastolic BP higher than 120.

            ➤ All patients with a systolic BP over 180 or a diastolic pressure over 120 (especially those who are symptomatic) should be transported.

   F. Cardiogenic Shock: see Chapter 15

 IV. **ASSESSMENT AND MANAGEMENT**

   A. See Chapter 9 for a summary of patient assessment.

   B. Any patient with chest pain or other signs and symptoms of a cardiac emergency should be considered a high transport priority.

   C. Consider pharmacology interventions, including oxygen, aspirin, and nitroglycerine (follow local protocols).

D. Consider CPAP for CHF patients with significant respiratory distress.

E. Acquisition and transmission of a 12-lead ECG is an EMT skill. See illustration to review lead placement. Follow local protocol regarding 12-lead ECG acquisition.

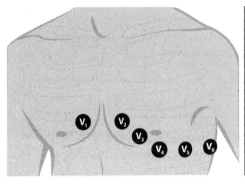

V₁	Fourth intercostal space to the right of the sternum
V₂	Fourth intercostal space to the left of the sternum
V₃	Directly between leads V₂ and V₄
V₄	Fifth intercostal space at mid-clavicular line
V₅	Level with V₄ at left anterior axillary line
V₆	Level with V₅ at left mid-axillary line (midpoint under armpit)

Figure 12-1: Lead Placement

V. SPECIAL CONSIDERATIONS

A. Automatic implantable cardioverter-defibrillators (AICD)

1. An AICD is like an AED but is placed under the skin and connected directly to the heart.

2. Energy level from AICD is much lower than an AED, so it presents minimal risk to providers.

3. Treat as you would any other patient; however, when applying an AED, avoid placing pads directly over device.

B. Pacemaker

1. An implanted device that helps regulate a patient's cardiac rate by serving as an artificial source of electrical impulses to stimulate the heart.

2. Patients with malfunctioning pacemaker often experience dizziness, weakness, bradycardia, and hypotension.

3. Treat as you would any other patient; however, if applying an AED, avoid placing pads directly over device.

C. Ventricular assist device (VAD)

1. A mechanical device that is placed inside a person's chest to replace the function of the ventricles for patients with a failing heart.

2. May be a temporary or permanent treatment.

3. Most VADs produce continuous flow, so the patient may not have a palpable pulse or measurable blood pressure.

4. Look for cable from abdominal wall connecting to the device.

5. SpO_2 may be inaccurate. Use mental status and skin condition to assess perfusion and oxygenation.

6. Patient and family will be knowledgeable about VAD and will have contact info for VAD coordinator. Consult the VAD coordinator for help.

7. Consult medical direction for appropriate destination.

8. Keep the batteries and controller with the patient.

9. Use the AED as you normally would; however, if applying an AED, avoid placing pads directly over the device (may need to place pads anterior/posterior).

10. Many VAD patients also have an implantable cardioverter-defibrillator (ICD).

 VI. RESUSCITATION

Note: Be sure to review the current American Heart Association Guidelines for Basic Life Support and Emergency Cardiovascular Care. Questions directly relating to these standards **will** be on your certification exam.

A. CPR Standards and Requirements

1. Candidates for the NREMT exam must have a current and valid CPR credential equivalent to the American Heart Association (AHA) Basic Life Support (BLS).

2. The current AHA BLS Provider Manual provides the standards for CPR and emergency cardiovascular care that will be included on the NREMT exam.

B. Highlights of AHA BLS Guidelines

1. Emphasis is on high-quality compressions.

2. Use of CAB approach for unresponsive patients.

3. Rate of compression: 10–20/minute.

4. Depth of compression

    i.   Adults: 2 to 2.4 inches

    ii. Children & infants: ⅓ the depth of the chest (approximately 2 inches and 1.5 inches, respectively)

5. Compression to ventilation ratio

    i.   Adults: always 30:2

    ii. Single rescuer: always 30:2

    iii. Children & infants (two-rescuer): 15:2

    iv. Neonates: 3:1

6. Allow full chest recoil between compressions.

7. Minimize interruptions in chest compressions.

8. No hyperventilation!

9. Automated external defibrillator

    i.   Apply the AED as soon as possible and if safe to do so.

    ii. Follow prompts provided by AED.

    iii. Pediatric pads typically placed anterior/posterior.

10. Special situations

    i.   Pregnant patients

        ➤ Prone to hypoxia, so aggressive airway management and oxygenation is indicated.

        ➤ Provide continuous lateral uterine displacement for pregnant patients in cardiac arrest.

    ii. Hypothermic patients should typically only be shocked once by AED prior to transport. Follow local protocol.

    iii. Mechanical CPR devices provide consistent rate and depth of compressions; however, there is no current evidence that these devices improve survival rates compared to manual CPR. Follow local protocol regarding use of mechanical CPR devices.

11. Withholding resuscitation

   i. Confirm DNR status when applicable and possible.

   ii. Follow local protocol regarding withholding or terminating resuscitation efforts.

   iii. Consult medical direction with any questions.

C. Automated external defibrillators (AEDs)

1. Types of AED

   i. Semi-automatic AEDs: These AEDs have a button to deliver a shock. Semi-automatic AEDs are used by rescuers.

   ii. Fully-automatic AEDs: These AEDs do **not** have a shock button, they will automatically shock the patient if a shockable rhythm is detected. Fully-automatic AEDs are typically used by lay rescuers with minimal training.

2. Indications for the AED

   i. Pulseless adults and infants (over 28 days old)

   ii. Adults and children 8 years of age and older: adult AED pads

   iii. Infants and children under 8 years of age: pediatric AED pads

3. Contraindications

   i. Unsafe conditions

   ii. Any patient with a pulse

   iii. Neonates (birth to one month)

4. AED operation

   i. Determine unresponsiveness, check pulse, begin chest compressions and attach AED as soon as possible.

   ii. Turn on power and follow the verbal and visual prompts.

   iii. Apply AED

   ➤ Expose chest and remove any medication patches as needed.

> ➤ Move jewelry, such as a necklace, to the side—but do not waste time removing.

> ➤ Dry chest if wet and shave excess chest hair if needed.

> ➤ Apply pads according to manufacturer's instructions.

> ➤ Avoid placing pads directly over pacemaker, implanted defibrillator, VAD, etc.

    iv. Deliver shock as indicated and when safe to do so (ensure everyone is clear).

    v. Resume CPR immediately.

    vi. AED should automatically reanalyze after 2 minutes of CPR.

    vii. Initiate transport according to local protocol.

5. Special situations

    i. AEDs may not deliver a shock in a moving ambulance.

    ii. Adult AED pads can be used on a pediatric patient when absolutely necessary; however, pediatric pads cannot be used on an adult patient.

VI. SPECIAL PATIENTS

A. Pediatrics

1. ***Important:*** Unresponsive pediatric patients with a pulse lower than 60 require CPR.

2. Bradycardia in pediatric patients is a sign of hypoxia until proven otherwise.

B. Elderly patients

1. The geriatric patient population is growing rapidly.

2. Elderly patients are at increased risk of ACS, CHF, and aortic aneurysm.

PRACTICE QUESTIONS

Answers on page 385.

1. Which of the following statements regarding unstable angina is correct? (Select the TWO answer options that apply.)

   A. Unstable angina is typically resolved by rest.

   B. Unstable angina is usually caused by exertion or stress.

   C. Unstable angina is an example of acute coronary syndrome.

   D. Unstable angina is unpredictable.

   E. Unstable angina is not an indication for nitroglycerine.

2. Which of the following are common signs and symptoms of congestive heart failure? (Select the THREE answer options that apply.)

   A. JVD

   B. pulmonary edema

   C. abdominal distention

   D. pedal edema

   E. flat neck veins

   F. hyperactivity

3. Your patient is on a ventricular assist device. The patient is likely suffering from which of the following?

   A. pulmonary embolism

   B. heart failure

   C. hypertensive crisis

   D. mild angina

4. What is the compression to ventilation ration for two-rescuer child CPR?

   A. 3:1

   B. 5:1

   C. 15:2

   D. 30:2

5. The CAB approach to assessment should be used for

   A. unresponsive patients.

   B. all patients.

   C. pediatric patients only.

   D. alert patients.

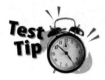

Test Tip

Questions on the NREMT exam will likely focus on:

- High-frequency tasks that EMTs perform routinely based on the NREMT EMS Practice Analysis

- High-risk tasks that are likely to cause harm if not performed competently by the EMT

Stroke, Seizures, and Syncope

I. TERMS TO KNOW

A. **Atherosclerosis:** Build-up of plaques in the arteries.

B. **GCS:** Glasgow Coma Scale.

C. **Stroke:** Death to brain tissue due to an interruption in blood flow.

D. **Syncope:** Fainting spell.

E. **Transient ischemic attack:** A brief episode of neurological dysfunction resulting from an interruption in the blood supply to the brain.

II. PATHOPHYSIOLOGY

A. Stroke is the fifth leading cause of death in the United States.

B. Most strokes are ischemic, not hemorrhagic.

C. Hypotension is the most common cause of syncope.

III. STROKE

A. A stroke is death to brain tissue due to an interruption in blood flow.

1. Also called a cerebrovascular accident or brain attack.

2. In most cases, modern treatments can significantly reduce the amount of damage and disability if initiated in time.

B. Ischemic stroke

1. Most strokes are caused by ischemia due to atherosclerosis (buildup of plaque in the arteries), which compromises blood flow to the brain.

2. About 87% of strokes are ischemic.

C. Hemorrhagic strokes

1. Caused by bleeding within the brain (about 13% of all strokes).

2. Intracerebral bleeding robs brain of oxygen delivery and can apply pressure to brain tissue.

3. Treatment options more limited with hemorrhagic strokes and they are more often fatal compared to ischemic strokes.

D. Signs and symptoms of stroke

1. Slurred speech

2. Facial droop

3. Headache

4. Unilateral (one-sided) weakness or paralysis

5. Difficulty walking

6. Vision problems

7. Altered mentation

E. Stroke Assessments

1. Stroke assessments (stroke scales) are designed to identify the probability of a stroke.

2. When performed correctly, they are highly accurate.

3. Follow local protocol regarding which stroke scale to use. A stroke assessment should be performed on any patient you suspect may be having a stroke.

    i. Cincinnati Prehospital Stroke Scale (CPSS)

        ➤ Facial droop

           — Ask the patient to smile.

           — Facial droop is indicative of possible stroke.

> Arm drift

— Ask patient to close eyes while holding arms out, palms up.

— Arm drift is indicative of possible stroke.

> Slurred speech

— Ask the patient to repeat a given sentence.

— Slurred speech or incorrect word choice is indicative of a stroke.

> CPSS is greater than 70% accurate with one abnormal finding and over 85% accurate with three abnormal findings.

ii. BE-FAST Stroke Assessment

> **Balance:** Did patient experience sudden loss of balance or ability to walk?

> **Eyes:** Any acute changes in vision?

> **Facial droop**

> **Arm drift**

> **Speech**

> **Time:** when did symptoms first appear?

iii. Los Angeles Prehospital Stroke Screen (LPSS)

> Similar to CPSS, but more in-depth.

> Requires nine assessments (detailed below) instead of three.

F. Assessment and Management of Stroke Patient

1. See summary of patient assessment in Chapter 9.

2. It is critical to determine the exact onset of stroke-like symptoms whenever possible.

3. Any patient with signs or symptoms of a possible stroke should be considered a high transport priority. Do **not** delay transport of a suspected stroke patient.

4. Suspected stroke patients should be transported to an approved stroke center per local protocol. Notify stroke center so stroke team can prepare.

5. Protect the patient from further harm during movement and transport.

6. Communicate with patient even if they seem unaware of their surroundings.

7. Follow American Heart Association guidelines and local protocol regarding oxygen administration for stroke patients.

8. Avoid tunnel vision. Be aware of conditions that can mimic a stroke, such as hypoglycemia, head injury, postictal state.

9. Obtain Glasgow Coma Scale (GCS) score. Do **not** delay transport to determine GCS.

Table 13-1 Glasgow Coma Scale (GCS)

Eye opening	Spontaneous	4
	To speech To pain	3
	None	2
		1
Verbal response	Alert and oriented	5
	Confused	4
	Inappropriate	3
	Incomprehensible	2
	None	1
Motor response	Obeys commands	6
	Localizes pain	5
	Withdraws from pain	4
	Abnormal flexion	3
	Abnormal extension	2
	None	1
	Total Score:	Min. 3/Max. 15

Note: A lower GCS score indicates a higher likelihood of brain injury and the need for rapid intervention and transport.

Note: Your documentation should include the following:

- Time of onset of symptoms
- GCS score
- Results of stroke assessment tool used
- Any changes during care

IV. TRANSIENT ISCHEMIC ATTACK (TIA)

A. TIAs have the same presentation as a stroke; however, the signs and symptoms self-correct within about 24 hours with no permanent brain damage.

B. TIAs are sometimes called "mini-strokes" by patients.

C. About one-third of TIA patients will have a stroke within one year.

D. Treat all patients with signs and symptoms of a stroke or TIA as stroke patients (high-priority transport to an appropriate facility).

V. SEIZURES

A. Seizures are caused by disorganized electrical activity in the brain.

B. Types of seizures

1. Generalized seizures

   i. Also called tonic-clonic or grand mal seizures.

   ii. Patient is unresponsive and experiences full-body convulsions.

   iii. Patient may experience temporary respiratory arrest.

2. Absence seizures

   i. Also called petit mal seizures.

   ii. Patient unable to interact with surrounding environment, but there are no convulsions.

3. Partial seizures

   i. Simple partial seizures

      ➤ No convulsions or change in LOC

      ➤ Possible twitching or sensory changes

   ii. Complex partial seizures

      ➤ Altered LOC

      ➤ Isolated twitching and sensory changes possible

4. Status epilepticus

    i.   Generalized seizure lasting longer than 5 minutes or having more than one seizure within 5 minutes or without regaining consciousness between seizures.

    ii.   Dangerous seizure activity that can lead to permanent brain damage and death.

5. Phases of a generalized tonic-clonic (grand mal) seizure

    i.   Aura phase

        ➤ Warning stage

        ➤ Some patients sense they are about to have a seizure.

    ii.   Tonic phase

        ➤ Loss of consciousness

        ➤ Muscle rigidity, spasms

        ➤ Possible respiratory paralysis

        ➤ May bite tongue, cheek, or become incontinent

    iii.   Clonic phase

        ➤ Jerking movement

        ➤ Usually lasts under 3 minutes

    iv.   Postictal phase

        ➤ Recovery phase

        ➤ Patient begins breathing

        ➤ Will remain unconscious for several minutes, then gradually wake up

6. Causes of Seizures

    i.   Seizures can be caused by congenital problems, trauma, drugs/alcohol, brain injury, tumors, diabetic emergencies, epilepsy (brain disorder), fever, infection, medications, poisoning, stroke, and more.

    ii.   Failure to take seizure medication as prescribed is one of the most common causes of seizures.

    iii.   Febrile (fever) seizures are common in pediatric patients.

iv. AEIOU-TIPS: mnemonic used to recall common causes of altered mental status

  ➤ Alcohol, Acids/Alkalis

  ➤ Epilepsy, Endocrine (such as hyper- or hypoglycemia)

  ➤ Insulin

  ➤ Opiates, Overdose

  ➤ Uremia (kidney failure), Underdose (e.g., did not take seizure medications)

  ➤ Trauma

  ➤ Increased ICP, Infection

  ➤ Poisoning, Psychiatric

  ➤ Seizures, Syncope, Shock, Stroke

Note: You should always assess SpO_2 and blood glucose on any patient with an altered LOC.

7. Recognizing and Managing Seizures

  i. In most cases, the seizure activity will be over by the time you arrive. You will often find the patient in the postictal phase.

  ii. Place unresponsive patients on their side in case of vomiting.

  iii. Question bystanders.

  iv. Assess for incontinence, trauma to tongue/cheek.

  v. Assess SpO_2 and blood glucose.

  vi. Allow the patient time to become alert and oriented before obtaining history.

  vii. Be prepared for additional seizure activity.

  viii. If patient is still actively seizing, protect from harm.

VI. SYNCOPE

A. Syncope is fainting. Typically caused by temporary loss of blood flow to the brain.

B. There are many causes of syncope, including irregular heartbeat, hypotension, neurological problems, stress, diabetes, pregnancy.

C. Patients typically regain consciousness quickly.

D. Obtain thorough history, assess SpO$_2$, blood glucose.

E. When in doubt, encourage treatment and transport.

 VII. HEADACHE

A. Headaches have many causes, some are serious (stroke, aneurysm, hypertensive crisis, brain tumor, trauma, meningitis).

B. Headache "red flags." The following accompanying conditions indicate a possible life-threatening condition:

1. Severe headache ("This is the worst headache I've ever had")
2. Sudden onset of severe headache
3. Altered mentation
4. Older than 50 years of age
5. Immunocompromised
6. Hypertension
7. Fever
8. Stiff neck
9. Vision changes
10. Neurological impairment (signs of a stroke)
11. Recent trauma

 VIII. SPECIAL PATIENT POPULATIONS

A. Pediatric patients

1. Febrile seizures due to viral infection are the most common cause of seizures in pediatric patients. Febrile seizures are due to sudden onset of high fever.

2. Febrile seizures are usually well-tolerated by pediatric patients; however, always transport a pediatric patient who has experienced a seizure.

B. Elderly patients

1. Brain shrinks with age, increasing risk of brain injury from even minor trauma.

2. Over 70% of strokes occur in patients over age 65.

3. Severe headaches in patients over age 50 should be taken seriously.

4. New-onset seizures in elderly patients is not uncommon.

C. Trauma patients

1. Consider need for spinal motion restriction. Follow local protocol.

2. Be alert for signs of traumatic brain injury. See Chapter 18 for additional information.

Note: Most people have experienced a headache. Most don't call 9-1-1 for it. If your patient has a headache bad enough to call 9-1-1, it should be taken seriously. Pay special attention to headache "red flags."

PRACTICE QUESTIONS
Answers on page 386.

1. Death to brain tissue due to an interruption of blood flow is known as

A. a transient ischemic attack.

B. a stroke.

C. myocardial infarction.

D. syncope.

2. Which of the following are part of the Cincinnati Prehospital Stroke Scale? (Select the THREE answer options that apply.)

   A. blood pressure

   B. slurred speech

   C. GCS score

   D. arm drift

   E. facial droop

   F. blood glucose

3. Your patient is unresponsive and experiencing full-body convulsions. The patient is presenting with

   A. generalized seizures.

   B. absence seizures.

   C. petit mal seizures.

   D. simple partial seizures.

4. Which of the following types of seizures presents the greatest risk of permanent brain damage or death?

   A. complex partial seizure

   B. petit mal seizures

   C. febrile seizure

   D. status epilepticus

5. Which of the following is a headache "red flag"? (Select the TWO answer options that apply.)

   A. patients over age 50

   B. a history of sinus infections

   C. patients on OTC NSAIDs

   D. hypertension

   E. gradual onset of pain

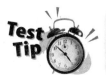
Test Tip

Often, you can anticipate the correct answer to a question before reading the answer choices. When you see an answer choice similar to what you envisioned, it's probably the correct answer.

PART V

SHOCK, TRAUMA, AND ENVIRONMENTAL EMERGENCIES

REVIEW PLUS
END-OF-CHAPTER PRACTICE

Trauma Overview

I. TERMS TO KNOW

A. **Index of suspicion:** Awareness and concern for potential injury.

B. **Kinetic energy:** Energy from motion.

C. **MVC:** Motor vehicle collision.

D. **SRS:** Safety restraint system.

E. **TBI:** Traumatic brain injury.

II. PATHOPHYSIOLOGY OF TRAUMA

A. Trauma is the leading cause of death up to age 45 and the fourth leading cause of death overall.

B. Traumatic brain injury is the leading cause of trauma-related deaths.

III. INTRO TO MECHANISM OF INJURY (MOI) AND KINEMATICS OF TRAUMA

A. Mechanism of injury refers to the way traumatic injuries occur. Examples:

1. Blunt trauma vs. penetrating trauma

2. Low velocity vs. high velocity

3. Isolated vs. multisystem

B. Kinematic energy comes from an object in motion

    1. Kinetic energy = ½ mass × velocity²

    2. *Note:* Velocity plays a much bigger role than mass.

C. Applying MOI and kinematics to EMS

    1. Understanding the MOI can help predict injury patterns.

    2. Index of suspicion: Ability to predict what types of injuries are likely based on the MOI.

    3. Example: Your patient was in a vehicle that was struck from behind. Assessment of the MOI would help you determine that spinal injury is more likely than lower extremity injury.

    4. EMS providers don't diagnose; however, they have the latitude to rule in the possibility of injury based on three key factors:

        i. The MOI (Example: shooting)

        ii. The anatomical findings (Example: sucking chest wound)

        iii. The physiological presentation of the patient (Example: absent lung sounds)

D. Blunt trauma

    1. Blunt trauma is non-penetrating trauma due to impact with a firm surface or object.

    2. Falls and motor vehicle collisions are common causes of blunt trauma.

    3. More traumatic deaths are due to blunt trauma than penetrating trauma.

E. Penetrating trauma

    1. Low velocity penetrating trauma

        i. Example: knife, pencil, rebar, etc.

        ii. Injury follows path of the penetrating object.

    2. Medium velocity penetrating trauma

        i. Example: most handguns.

        ii. Injury pattern can be unpredictable due to ricochet, shrapnel.

3. High velocity penetrating trauma

  i. Example: assault rifle.

  ii. Injury path can be many times larger than projectile due to cavitation (formation of space within body).

IV. INJURY MECHANISMS

A. Motor vehicle collisions (MVC)

  1. Types of MVCs

  i. Head-on collisions

  ➤ Occupants can go up and over, or down and under, the dashboard.

  ➤ Head, spinal, chest, abdomen, pelvic, and lower extremity injuries are common.

  ➤ Unrestrained passengers are more likely to be ejected.

  ii. Rear-impact collisions

  ➤ C-spine injuries are common, including whiplash.

  ➤ Rear-impact collisions typically cause hyperextension of the neck.

  iii. Lateral-impact collisions ("T-bone")

  ➤ Injuries along the side of impact are common.

  ➤ Example: Drivers struck on driver's side are at higher risk of spleen injury than passengers struck on the passenger side.

  iv. Rollovers

  ➤ Injury patterns are not predictable.

  ➤ High risk of multisystem trauma and occupant ejection.

Note: Let's look at a scenario where you are caring for the restrained driver of a vehicle that rolled several times. She is your only patient. During your walk-around of the vehicle, you observe that the passenger-side windshield is starred and the passenger airbag deployed. Several yards from the vehicle, you find a car seat with extensive damage. Do you only have one patient? This is one example of why it is important to assess the MOI.

     v.   Rotational spins

       ➤ High risk of multisystem trauma, including spinal injury.

       ➤ Less common than rear impact and lateral impact.

2. Importance of assessing vehicle damage

   i.   Assessing the vehicle helps you better understand the MOI and amount of force (kinetic energy) the patient was exposed to.

   ii. Example: Your index of suspicion for serious injury should go up if the vehicle the patient was in suffered extensive damage.

3. Assessing MOI

   i.   What did the vehicle hit or get hit by?

   ii. What speed was the impact?

   iii. Where is the damage to the vehicle, and how extensive is it?

   iv. How much intrusion was there into the occupant compartment?

   v. Did airbags deploy?

   vi. Were the occupants restrained properly?

   vii. Are any windows broken?

   viii. What is the condition of the steering column, steering wheel, dashboard, etc.?

4. The three collisions of an MVC

   i.   First collision: The vehicle strikes an object.

   ii. Second collision: The occupants strike the interior of the vehicle or the safety restraint system (SRS).

   iii. Third collision: Internal organs strike the internal structures of the body.

5. Safety restraint system

   i.   The SRS in modern vehicles includes lap belts, shoulder harness, and air bags.

   ii. The SRS can reduce deceleration injuries caused by second and third collisions.

6. High-risk MVCs

   i.   Rollover accidents.

   ii. Any MVC with occupant ejection.

      iii. Death of another occupant in the same vehicle.

      iv. Pedestrians, cyclists, and motorcyclists struck by vehicles.

      v. MVC resulting in extensive damage to the vehicle.

      vi. Damage that intrudes into the occupant compartment.

B. Fall injuries

  1. You must determine three things:

      i. How far did the patient fall?

      ii. What surface did the patient land on?

      iii. How did the patient land?

  2. High-risk fall injuries

      i. Ground-level falls in elderly patients (age 65 or older)

      ii. Falls of 20 feet or more in adults and 10 feet or more in pediatric patients

      iii. Any fall with resulting loss of consciousness or signs of multisystem trauma or shock

F. Blast injuries

  1. Primary blast injuries: caused by pressure wave of the blast.

  2. Secondary blast injuries: caused by flying debris.

  3. Tertiary blast injuries: caused by being thrown against a stationary object.

  4. Quaternary blast injuries: everything else, such as burns, toxic fumes.

V. TRAUMA TRIAGE

A. Indications for air medical transport

  1. Extended extrication time

  2. Distance from appropriate hospital destination over about 20 miles

  3. No other ALS providers available

  4. Multiple patients, mass casualty incidents

  5. Delay of ground transport

B. Hospital destination

1. High-priority trauma patients should be seen at a Level 1 Trauma Center. Follow local protocol.

2. Not all Level 1 Trauma Centers are equipped to receive pediatric patients. Follow local protocol.

C. Trauma center designations

1. Level 1 Trauma Centers: Capable of handling all types of trauma 24/7. Trauma teams are on-site. Facility has emergency surgery capability and trauma ICU.

2. Level 2 Trauma Center: Capable of stabilizing trauma patients and transferring them to a Level 1 Trauma Center as needed.

3. Level 3 and 4 Trauma Centers: Limited services and ability to stabilize trauma patients.

Note: Most Level 1 Trauma Centers will expect you to report the patient's Glasgow Coma Scale (GCS) score during your report to the trauma team.

Table 14-1 Glasgow Coma Scale (GCS)

Eye opening	Spontaneous	4
	To speech To pain	3
	None	2
		1
Verbal response	Alert and oriented	5
	Confused	4
	Inappropriate	3
	Incomprehensible	2
	None	1
Motor response	Obeys commands	6
	Localizes pain	5
	Withdraws from pain	4
	Abnormal flexion	3
	Abnormal extension	2
	None	1
	Total Score:	Min. 3/Max. 15

Note: A lower GCS score indicates a higher likelihood of brain injury and the need for rapid intervention and transport.

VI. SPECIAL PATIENTS

A. At-risk populations

   1. 97% of women with mental illness who are homeless have experienced severe physical and/or sexual trauma.

   2. Transgender individuals are four times more likely to be the victims of violent crime.

B. Pediatrics

   1. Most pediatric trauma-related deaths are due to motor vehicle collisions.

   2. Drowning is the leading cause of injury-related deaths in children 1–4 years old.

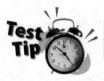

Test Tip If flashcards are a learning tool that works well for you, be sure to study a few of them every day. Repetition is essential. Repetition is essential.

PRACTICE QUESTIONS
Answers on page 387.

1. Which of the following is true regarding rear-impact MVCs?

   A. Injuries along the left side of the driver's body are common.

   B. Occupants are likely to go down and under the dash.

   C. Neck injuries due to hyperextension are common.

   D. Injury patterns are not predictable with rear-impact collisions.

2. The risk of occupant ejection is highest with

   A. a rollover.

   B. a lateral impact.

   C. a head-on collision.

   D. a rotational spin.

3. Your patient was a passenger in a vehicle that struck a tree. Which of the following is considered the "third collision" based on this mechanism?

   A. The vehicle's impact with the tree.

   B. The patient's internal organs striking the internal structure of the body.

   C. The patient's collision with the vehicle or seat belt and airbag.

   D. The vehicle's collision with other objects as it bounces off the tree.

4. Which of the following are considered high-risk fall injuries? (Select the TWO answer options that apply.)

   A. All falls in patients over age 35.

   B. Falls greater than 20 feet.

   C. Any fall resulting in loss of consciousness.

   D. Falls greater than 5 feet in pediatric patients.

   E. Falls without signs of shock.

5. Your patient has injuries resulting from the pressure wave of an explosion. These injuries are considered

   A. primary blast injuries.

   B. secondary blast injuries.

   C. tertiary blast injuries.

   D. quaternary blast injuries.

Bleeding and Shock

I. TERMS TO KNOW

A. **Angioedema:** Swelling under the tissue, often in the face or tongue.

B. **Compensated shock:** Early shock where the body still maintains adequate perfusion.

C. **Evisceration:** An open abdominal wound with internal organs protruding.

D. **Decompensated shock:** Late shock where the body can no longer maintain adequate perfusion.

E. **Hemorrhage:** Bleeding.

F. **Poikilothermia:** An inability to regulate core body temperature.

G. **Urticaria:** Hives.

II. SHOCK

A. Pathophysiology of Shock

1. Perfusion is the adequate circulation of oxygenated blood throughout the body. Perfusion is required to maintain homeostasis.

2. Shock (hypoperfusion) is inadequate tissue perfusion. The tissues and organs of the body are not getting the oxygenated blood flow from the circulatory system that is needed to function properly.

3. Shock is typically caused by a problem with the "pump, pipes, or fluid." This means shock is due to problems with the heart, the blood vessels, or the blood/plasma. This is known as the Perfusion Triangle.

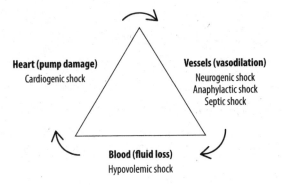

Figure 15-1: Perfusion Triangle

B. Stages of Shock

1. Compensated (early) shock

    i.   The body's defense mechanisms are still able to compensate for the problem.

    ii. Defense mechanisms include peripheral vasoconstriction and increased heart rate.

2. Decompensated (late or progressive) shock

    i.   The body is no longer able to compensate for the problem.

    ii. Blood pressure begins to fall.

Note: This is a critical concept: The telltale characteristic of decompensated shock is falling blood pressure leading to hypotension.

3. Irreversible (terminal) shock

    i.   Rapid cardiovascular collapse (irreversible hypotension)

    ii. Non-survivable

C. The Shock Cycle

1. The shock cycle illustrates the physiologic changes that occur during shock.

2. Patients enter the shock cycle at various points depending on the type of shock, but then all patients continue the same spiral until recovery or death.

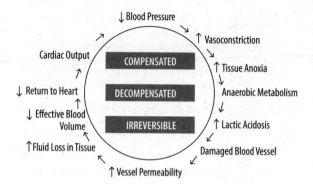

Figure 15-2: Shock Cycle

D. The body's compensatory mechanisms for shock

1. Tachycardia

    i.   If there is a loss of blood or plasma, the brain will increase rate and force of cardiac contraction to increase BP.

    ii. Certain medications can interfere with this process.

2. Peripheral vasoconstriction

    i.   The brain will trigger peripheral vasoconstriction to increase BP and prioritize blood flow to vital organs (brain, heart, lungs, kidneys).

    ii. Pediatric patients vasoconstrict well, which can mask the signs of shock.

    iii. Elderly patients do not typically vasoconstrict well, limiting their ability to compensate.

3. Increased respirations to combat hypoxia.

4. *Note:* Falling BP is a **late** sign of shock. Hypotension indicates that the body's defense mechanisms are failing.

    i.   If the patient has a low BP, they are **not** in compensated shock.

    ii. Treat all hypotensive shock patients as a high transport priority.

      iii. Pediatric patients can maintain their BP until about half of their blood volume has been lost. Do **not** wait for hypotension to begin aggressively treating a pediatric patient for shock.

E. Types of Shock

  1. Cardiogenic shock (pump problem)

      i. Heart muscle cannot pump effectively, causing a backup of fluid, pulmonary edema, and hypotension.

      ii. Most common cause is a significant myocardial infarction.

      iii. Not common and only about 50% of patients survive.

      iv. Signs and symptoms: hypotension, probable cardiac history, chest pain, dyspnea, pulmonary edema, altered LOC.

  2. Obstructive shock (obstruction of blood flow through the cardiovascular system)

      i. Cardiac tamponade ("pericardial tamponade")

        ➤ Fluid accumulates in pericardial sac and compresses the heart.

        ➤ Signs and symptoms: jugular vein distention JVD, narrowing pulse pressure (hypotension), muffled heart tones.

Note: The classic triad of findings for cardiac tamponade (JVD, hypotension, muffled heart tones) is called Beck's triad.

      ii. Tension pneumothorax

        ➤ Air enters the chest cavity due to lung injury or sucking chest wound. Accumulating pressure compresses the lungs and great vessels.

        ➤ Signs and symptoms: respiratory distress, diminished or absent lung sounds, JVD, poor BVM compliance, tracheal deviation toward unaffected side (this is a **late** sign).

      iii. Pulmonary embolism

        ➤ Occurs when one or more arteries in the lungs become blocked by a blood clot.

> ➤ The blood clot likely traveled from elsewhere in the body, through the right side of the heart, and into a pulmonary artery.

> ➤ Signs and symptoms: dyspnea, anxiety, chest pain, cough, cyanosis.

3. Distributive shock

  i. Distributive shock is primarily a problem with the blood vessels ("pipe problem").

  ii. Distributive shock causes widespread vasodilation, leading to relative hypovolemia and hypotension.

  iii. Anaphylactic shock (anaphylaxis)

  > ➤ Life-threatening allergic reaction due to

  >   — Systemic vasodilation (hypotension)

  >   — Widespread vessel permeability (fluid leakage)

  >   — Bronchoconstriction

  > ➤ Causes

  >   — Foods: nuts, milk, fish, shellfish, eggs, wheat, some fruit

  >   — Medications: antibiotics, NSAIDs such as aspirin

  >   — Insects: bees, wasps, fire ants

  >   — Other: latex, exercise (not common)

  > ➤ Signs and symptoms

  >   — Cardiovascular: acute, severe hypotension

  >   — Respiratory: wheezing, respiratory failure

  >   — Skin: hives, edema, angioedema

Note: "Relative" hypovolemia means that there is not enough blood volume relative to the size of the vascular space. Distributive shock causes massive vasodilation resulting in relative hypovolemia and hypotension.

  iv. Neurogenic shock

  > ➤ Neurogenic shock is usually caused by spinal cord injury (C1–C5). Less common causes include tumors, pressure on the spinal cord, spina bifida.

➤ Widespread vasodilation causes hypotension and relative hypovolemia.

➤ Neurogenic shock disrupts normal communication pathways between the CNS and PNS. This interferes with the body's normal compensatory mechanisms, such as tachycardia and peripheral vasoconstriction.

Note: Critical concept: patients in neurogenic shock will not likely present with the tachycardia and pale, cool, clammy skin you find in other forms of shock. Neurogenic shock patients **will** be hypotensive.

➤ Signs and symptoms

— MOI indicative of possible spinal cord injury

— Severe hypotension

— Warm skin, normal color (neurogenic shock patients can't vasoconstrict normally)

— Heart rate normal or bradycardic (injury prevents stimulation of heart rate)

— Paralysis possible depending on location and severity of injury

— Respiratory insufficiency or paralysis

— Priapism in males (persistent, painful, penile erection)

v. Septic shock

➤ Shock due to severe infection leading to vasodilation and fluid loss from vascular space.

➤ Blood vessels do not constrict well during septic shock.

➤ More common in people who have been hospitalized.

➤ Signs and symptoms

— Severe hypotension

— Fever, chills, weakness

— Recent hospitalization, illness, surgery

— Altered LOC

— Tachypnea

— Pale, cool, clammy skin

— Loss of appetite, poor fluid intake

vi. Psychogenic shock

> ➤ Psychogenic shock is fainting (syncope) caused by acute, temporary, widespread vasodilation.

> ➤ Does **not** typically cause sustained inadequate tissue perfusion.

> ➤ *Note:* Psychogenic shock is just one cause of syncope. There are many other causes, some of them serious.

vii. Hypovolemic shock

> ➤ Hypovolemic shock is a fluid problem. It can be caused by loss of whole blood (hemorrhage) or due to vomiting, dehydration, diarrhea, burn injury, etc.

> ➤ *Note:* Hemorrhagic shock is a form of hypovolemic shock; however, not all hypovolemic shock is due to hemorrhage.

> ➤ Pediatric and elderly patients are at higher risk of hypovolemic shock due to dehydration.

> ➤ Signs and symptoms

> > — Trauma with hemorrhage or suspected internal bleeding

> > — Vomiting, diarrhea

> > — Altered LOC

> > — Tachycardia

> > — Pale, cool, clammy skin

> > — Weak peripheral pulses

> > — Hypotension (late sign)

F. Signs and Symptoms of Shock

1. Early signs and symptoms

   i. *Note:* Many of the early signs and symptoms of shock are the result of the body's attempt to compensate and protect itself.

   ii. Altered LOC (restless, anxious, irritable). This should be considered an indication of possible early hypoxia.

   iii. Tachycardia (not with neurogenic shock)

      iv. Pale, cool, clammy skin (not with neurogenic shock below level of injury)

      v. Weak peripheral pulses (peripheral vasoconstriction)

      vi. Increased respiratory rate

      vii. Thirst

      viii. Possible delayed capillary refill (over 2 seconds) in pediatric patients

  2. Late signs and symptoms

      i. Falling blood pressure (eventually hypotension)

      ii. Irregular breathing

      iii. Mottling or cyanosis

      iv. Absent peripheral pulses

      v. Decreased LOC

  3. Remember, the presentation of neurogenic shock is unique

      i. Skin is usually warm, flushed.

      ii. Heart rate is often normal or bradycardic.

      iii. Paralysis, including respiratory paralysis, could be immediate.

G. Managing Shock (the five fundamental interventions)

  1. Control bleeding.

  2. Place patient supine when possible.

      i. Pregnant patients need to be tilted toward left side to prevent supine hypotensive syndrome.

      ii. Some shock patients (cardiogenic or obstructive) will not tolerate being placed supine.

  3. High-flow oxygen.

  4. Prevent heat loss.

  5. Rapid transport.

H. Special Patient Populations

  1. Pediatric patients often mask the signs of shock until they are close to circulatory collapse.

2. Pediatric and elderly patients are at increased risk of hypovolemic shock due to dehydration.

3. Always regard bradycardia in pediatric patients as a sign of hypoxia.

4. Remember, neurogenic shock does **not** present like other forms of shock.

5. Remember, elderly patients often do not compensate well for shock and can deteriorate quickly.

6. Suspect septic shock in any recently hospitalized or post-surgical patient with a fever.

7. In addition to standard shock management, anaphylactic patients also require epinephrine via auto-injector per local protocol.

III. BLEEDING

A. Types of bleeding

1. External

   i. May not be obvious if the patient isn't exposed for a thorough assessment.

   ii. Life-threatening external bleeding must be managed immediately.

Note: External bleeding is the single most preventable cause of traumatic death, but it must be managed quickly and aggressively.

2. Internal bleeding

   i. Harder to identify and more difficult to manage.

   ii. Presumption of internal bleeding based on signs & symptoms, MOI/NOI, and assessment:

      ➤ Blunt trauma

      ➤ History of internal bleeding

      ➤ Bruising

         — Cullen's sign: bruising around the umbilical region

         — Kehr's sign: left shoulder pain upon abdominal palpation when patient is supine with legs elevated (indicates a ruptured spleen)

> ➤ Hematoma

> ➤ Abdominal distention

> ➤ Blood stool? Dark, tarry stool

> ➤ Vomiting blood or "coffee-ground" emesis

> ➤ Signs and symptoms of shock

    iii. **Note:** Long bone fractures can lead to significant bleeding. Femur and pelvic fractures can cause life-threatening hemorrhage (1,000 mL from a single femur fracture and 1,500 mL from a pelvic fracture).

B. Sources of Bleeding

    1. Arteries: spurting, bright red blood

    2. Veins: steady flow of dark red blood

    3. Capillaries: slow, oozing bleeding with clearish fluid

C. Controlling External Bleeding

    1. Direct pressure. Use a sterile dressing if available.

    2. Tourniquet. If direct pressure does not control bleeding to an extremity, rapidly apply a tourniquet per local protocol.

        i. Apply proximal to the wound, distal to proximal joint and not directly over a joint.

        ii. Apply a second tourniquet, if needed, proximal to the first tourniquet.

        iii. Apply adequate pressure to control bleeding.

        iv. Record time of application and mark patient to indicate tourniquet has been applied.

        v. **Note:** Risk of permanent tissue damage from tourniquet is less than previously thought when applied correctly for periods under 2 hours.

    3. For bleeding from a location that doesn't allow tourniquet application, pack the wound using a hemostatic dressing, then apply pressure.

Note: No more PASG/MAST! Currently, there are **no** widely accepted indications for these devices, according to the American College of Surgeons and the American College of Emergency Physicians.

4. Special situations

   i. A junctional tourniquet is designed to control bleeding from inguinal and axilla areas where a standard tourniquet can't be applied.

   ii. A pelvic binder is designed to help stabilize a suspected pelvic fracture and reduce bleeding.

   iii. Epistaxis (nosebleed)

> Causes: trauma, hypertension, infection, allergy, foreign object

> Swallowing blood increases risk of vomiting.

> Can usually be controlled with firm pressure just below the bridge of the nose.

> Always assess the patient's blood pressure and question use of blood thinners.

> Consider sterile nasal-packing device, such as the Rhino Rocket. Follow local protocol.

   iv. Bleeding from nose or ears following head injury

> May be an indication of skull fracture.

> Apply loose dressing, but do not apply direct pressure due to risk of worsening traumatic brain injury.

D. Stop the Bleed

1. The American College of Surgeons "Stop the Bleed" course is recommended for all healthcare providers and lay rescuers.

2. Visit stopthebleed.org for additional information.

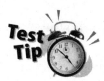
Test Tip

Patients who are hypotensive are in trouble. They should be treated as a high-transport priority. Remember the five fundamental interventions for managing shock.

PRACTICE QUESTIONS
Answers on page 387.

1. Which of the following best describes shock (hypoperfusion)?

   A. hypotension

   B. hypoxia

   C. inadequate tissue perfusion

   D. irreversible systemic collapse

2. Your trauma patient has lost an unknown amount of blood. He is alert, his pulse is slightly elevated, and his BP is normal. Based on this information, he is most likely experiencing which of the following?

   A. compensated shock

   B. anaphylactic shock

   C. decompensated shock

   D. neurogenic shock

3. Which of the following are indications of compensated shock? (Select the TWO answer options that apply.)

   A. tachycardia

   B. hypotension

   C. decreased LOC

   D. pale, cool, clammy skin

   E. irregular breathing

4. Which of the following correctly states how shock is experienced by pediatric patients?

   A. Pediatric patients rarely develop shock.

   B. Pediatric patients develop hypotension early.

   C. Pediatric patients mask the signs of shock until nearing circulatory collapse.

   D. Signs of shock with hypotension are not usually serious in pediatric patients.

5. Your patient presents with severe external bleeding to the arm. Direct pressure is not effectively controlling the bleeding. You should immediately do which of the following?

   A. Elevate the arm above the heart.

   B. Discontinue direct pressure and transport.

   C. Apply a pressure dressing.

   D. Apply a tourniquet.

Soft Tissue Injuries and Burns

I. TERMS TO KNOW

A. Contusion: A bruise.

B. Hematoma: A collection of blood beneath the skin.

C. Occlusive dressing: Airtight dressing.

D. Sprain: Ligament injury.

E. Strain: Muscle injury.

II. SOFT TISSUE INJURIES

A. Three types of soft tissue injuries

  1. Open injuries

    i. Types of open injuries

- Abrasion: a scrape
- Laceration: jagged cut
- Penetrating: puncture wound
- Incision: sharp, clean cut
- Avulsion: a flap of skin torn partially or completely loose
- Crush injury: may be open or closed
- Amputation: completely severed body part

      ii. Management of open soft tissue injuries

        ➤ Control bleeding as needed (see Chapter 15).

        ➤ Apply sterile dressing and bandage as needed.

2. Closed injuries

    i. Types of closed injuries

        ➤ Contusion: a bruise

        ➤ Hematoma: a collection of blood beneath the skin

        ➤ Crush injury: may be open or closed

    ii. Management of closed soft tissue injuries (RICES)

        ➤ **Rest**

        ➤ **I**ce

        ➤ **C**ompression (dressing)

        ➤ **E**levation

        ➤ **S**plinting

3. Special situations

    i. Compartment syndrome: Compression of nerves, vessels, and muscle in a closed space.

        ➤ Blood supply to tissues is compromised.

        ➤ Can cause permanent muscle damage, metabolic acidosis, renal failure, amputation, and death.

        ➤ Requires surgery to correct.

        ➤ The five "Ps" of compartment syndrome

           — Pain (severe pain is most common symptom)

           — Pallor (pale skin)

           — Paresthesia (numbness)

           — Pulselessness or faint pulse

           — Paralysis of affected area

        ➤ Poikilothermia is also a sign of compartment syndrome.

    ii. Open neck wounds and puncture wounds above the diaphragm should be covered with an occlusive dressing to prevent air embolism or sucking chest wound.

   iii. Evisceration: An open abdominal wound with internal organs (usually intestine) protruding.

- ➤ You must keep exposed organs moist and warm, and reduce the risk of infection.

- ➤ Cover with moist, sterile dressing.

- ➤ Cover moist dressing with occlusive dressing.

- ➤ Flex patient's legs to reduce contraction of abdominal muscles.

- ➤ Avoid placing the patient on his/her side.

- ➤ Treat for shock, including rapid transport.

   iv. Impaled objects

- ➤ Impaled objects should almost always be stabilized in place.

- ➤ Only two indications for removing an impaled object:

  - — The object creates an airway obstruction, inability to manage the airway or ventilate the patient.

  - — The object is in the chest and prevents CPR from being performed on a patient in cardiac arrest.

   v. Bite wounds

- ➤ All bite wounds that break the skin pose the risk of infection.

- ➤ Human bites are highly prone to infection. About one-third of all hand infections are due to human bites.

- ➤ Animal bites may lead to rabies. Notify animal control per local protocol.

- ➤ All bite wounds that break the skin should be seen by a physician due to the risk of infection and to determine whether a tetanus shot, rabies treatment, etc., is indicated.

Note: You can earn a certificate of completion in Advanced Burn Life Support (ABLS) online! Visit *www.ameriburn.org* for additional information.

III. BURN INJURIES

A. Pathophysiology

1. Most burns involve 10% or less of the patient's total body surface area.

2. 60% of thermal burns occur in children aged 5 and under.

3. 90% of burns can be managed without hospital admission.

4. Smoke detectors and other fire prevention strategies have reduced burn fatalities by 80%.

B. Life-threatening complications of burn injuries

1. Hypovolemia

2. Airway compromise

3. Hypothermia

4. Sepsis

C. The Five Factors of Burn Severity

1. Depth of the burn

    i. Superficial (first-degree) burn: epidermal damage only. Red and painful, but no blisters.

    ii. Partial thickness (second-degree) burn: epidermal and partial dermal injury. Painful and blisters present.

    iii. Full thickness (third-degree) burn: entire dermal layer destroyed. Dry, leathery skin (can be red, white, brown, charred) and no pain.

2. Amount of total body surface area (TBSA) burned

    i. Rule of nines: see Burn Center Referral Criteria (American Burn Association).

    ii. Rule of palm: the patient's hand (including fingers) equals about 1% of the patient's total TBSA.

3. Full-thickness burns to critical areas: hands, face, feet, genitalia, respiratory tract, and circumferential burns. (*Note:* Circumferential burns go all the way around a body part and can compromise distal perfusion as well as cause airway obstruction or respiratory failure.)

4. Associated trauma or preexisting medical conditions: associated trauma, poor health, and certain medications complicate the body's ability to handle a burn injury.

5. Age of patient: Patients under age 5 or over age 55 are at higher risk.

D. Severe Burn Injuries: see Burn Center Referral Criteria (American Burn Association). To learn more, visit *ameriburn.org/burnreferral.*

Guidelines for Burn Patient Referral

(Advice on Transfer and Consultation)

- These guidelines are designed to be used to aid in clinical decision making. If you have sustained a burn injury, please seek medical advice from a medical professional.
- Local and regional infrastructure, resources, and relationships may determine the necessity and timeliness of burn center referral.
- These guidelines are not meant to be definitive care recommendations. They may facilitate building the proper referral network within the local healthcare community.

	Immediate Consultation with Consideration for Transfer	Consultation Recommendation
Thermal Burns	• Full thickness burns • Partial thickness ≥10% TBSA* • Any deep partial or full thickness burns involving the face, hands, genitalia, feet, perineum, or over any joints • Patients with burns and other comorbidities • Patients with concomitant traumatic injuries • Poorly controlled pain	• Partial thickness burns <10% TBSA* • All potentially deep burns of any size
Inhalation Injury	• All patients with suspected inhalation injury	• Patients with signs of potential inhalation such as facial flash burns, singed facial hairs, or smoke exposure
Pediatrics (≤14 years, or <30 kg)	• All pediatric burns may benefit from burn center referral due to pain, dressing change needs, rehabilitation, patient/caregiver needs, or non-accidental trauma	
Chemical Injuries	• All chemical injuries	
Electrical Injuries	• All high voltage (≥1,000V) electrical injuries • Lightning injury	• Low voltage (<1,000V) electrical injuries should receive consultation and consideration for follow-up in a burn center to screen for delayed symptom onset and vision problems

Burn Severity Determination

SUPERFICIAL
- Dry, red, easily blanching, sometimes painful
- Example: Sunburn
- NOT counted in calculations of total burn surface area (TBSA)

SUPERFICIAL PARTIAL THICKNESS
- Moist, red, blanching, blisters, very painful
- Counted in calculations of total burn surface area (TBSA)

DEEP PARTIAL THICKNESS
- Drier, more pale, less blanching, less pain
- Counted in calculations of total burn surface area (TBSA)

FULL THICKNESS
- Dry, leathery texture, variable color (white, brown, black), loss of pin prick sensation
- Counted in calculations of total burn surface area (TBSA)

Percentage Total Body Surface Area (TBSA)

"RULE OF NINES"   "PALMAR METHOD"

Patient's entire palmar surface is approximately 1%

For more information visit **ameriburn.org/burnreferral**

Source: American Burn Association

E. Management of Thermal Burn Injuries

1. Stop the burning process. If the skin is still hot, the damage is ongoing. Apply moist, sterile burn sheet (cool water, **not** cold water and **never** ice) until the skin is no longer hot (3 to 5 minutes max), then apply a dry, sterile burn sheet and cover with a blanket to prevent heat loss. Don't forget to cover the head also to prevent heat loss.

2. Remove clothing that may be trapping heat. Do **not** peel off clothing melted onto the skin.

3. Remove jewelry (massive swelling is common).

4. Treat for shock and transport rapidly to an appropriate facility according to local protocol.

5. Burn injuries over 20% TBSA will result in systemic edema and increased risk of hypovolemic shock.

F. Special Situations

1. Inhalation injury

   i. Typically involves thermal burns in upper airway, or carbon monoxide (CO) poisoning, or chemical inhalation.

   ii. Signs and symptoms: altered mental status, stridor, dyspnea, coughing, wheezing, facial burns, hoarse voice, airway edema, singed facial hair or soot in the mouth. *Note:* Lack of facial burns does **not** rule out inhalation injury.

   iii. Any burn patient with signs of airway involvement requires high-flow oxygen and rapid transport.

   iv. Expect significant edema to develop over the next 24 to 48 hours.

   v. Carbon monoxide can be cleared from the bloodstream 3x faster with high-flow oxygen administration compared to room air.

2. Electrical burns

   i. Do **not** attempt to remove a patient from an electrical source without proper training.

   ii. Significant unseen injury may have occurred between entrance and exit wounds.

   iii. High risk of respiratory and cardiac arrest.

iv. All patients with electrical injury should be transported and evaluated by a physician.

3. Chemical burns

    i. Do **not** risk exposure without proper training. If safe to do so:

       ➤ Remove contaminated clothing, jewelry.

       ➤ Brush off any dry chemical.

       ➤ Irrigate exposed areas with copious amounts of water for at least 20 minutes (unless chemical is water-reactive).

       ➤ Avoid contaminating unaffected areas with runoff.

       ➤ Treat as thermal burn.

    ii. Eyes and respiratory system at high risk for injury from chemical exposure.

    iii. Hydrofluoric acid exposure

       ➤ Incidents are uncommon, but extremely dangerous and a potential hazard for rescuers.

       ➤ Hydrofluoric acid is an extremely strong acid found in glass etching, metal cleaning, rust removers, toilet bowl cleaners, metal polishes, and more.

       ➤ Topical exposure can rapidly cause significant burn injuries through all layers of the skin and into the bone. Inhalation or ingestion are often fatal.

       ➤ Apply 2.5% calcium gluconate gel for topical exposure (per local protocol).

4. Abuse

    i. Be alert for signs of abuse, particularly with pediatric patients, elderly patients, and special needs patients.

    ii. Older patients who are institutionalized, confused, or unable to communicate are at high risk of abuse.

    iii. Burn injuries account for about 10% of child abuse cases and 10% of admissions to Burn Centers.

    iv. Be alert for "classic dip" or "stocking-pattern burns" burns to feet, lower legs, buttocks, and genitalia.

       ➤ No splash marks

       ➤ Clear demarcation

       ➤ Unexplained or inconsistent explanation

v. Pediatric patients do **not** tolerate burn injuries well. They can become hypovolemic and hypothermic rapidly.

vi. Scalding burns are common in pediatric patients and usually preventable. The rule of palm often works better for estimating TBSA than the rule of nines.

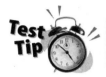

Test Tip

> **Important:** Isolated burn injuries do not cause the patient to have an altered LOC. If your burn patient has altered mentation, you should suspect other causes (hypoperfusion, head injury, hypoxia, hypoglycemia, inhalation injury, etc.).

PRACTICE QUESTIONS
Answers on page 388.

1. Your patient has a circumferential burn. This means that the burn

   A. goes all the way around a part of the body.

   B. covers more than 10% of the body.

   C. has damaged all layers of the skin.

   D. presents with a rounded burn pattern.

2. Which of the following burn injuries should be seen at a Burn Center? (Select the THREE answer options that apply.)

   A. All burns to pediatric patients.

   B. Partial thickness burns over 5% total body surface area.

   C. Electrical burns.

   D. Chemical burns.

   E. Burns to the lower back or buttocks.

   F. Burns with inhalation injury.

3. The patient's hand equals about

    A. 1% of the patient's total BSA.

    B. 2% of the patient's total BSA.

    C. 3% of the patient's total BSA.

    D. 4% of the patient's total BSA.

4. Which of the following soft tissue injuries can be open or closed?

    A. avulsion

    B. incision

    C. contusion

    D. crush injury

5. When should an impaled object be removed?

    A. never

    B. always

    C. when it prevents airway management

    D. when it is difficult to stabilize

Musculoskeletal Injuries

I. TERMS TO KNOW

A. **Crepitus:** Sound or feeling of fractured bone rubbing together.

B. **Dislocation:** Injury where a bone is displaced from a joint.

C. **Fracture:** Broken bone.

D. **Open fracture:** A fracture with a break in the skin.

E. **Pathologic fracture:** A fracture due to disease.

II. TYPES OF INJURIES

A. Fractures

   1. Open and closed fractures

      i.   Open fracture: a fracture with an associated open soft tissue injury

      ii. Closed fracture: a fracture where the skin is not broken

   2. Types of fractures (see Figure 17-1)

   3. Signs and symptoms of a fracture

      i.   Pain, tenderness

      ii. Swelling, deformity

      iii. Loss of function

      iv. Weak or absent distal pulses

     v.   Crepitus: the sound or feeling of fractured bone rubbing together

    4. Pathologic fractures: fractures due to disease, such as osteoporosis or cancer

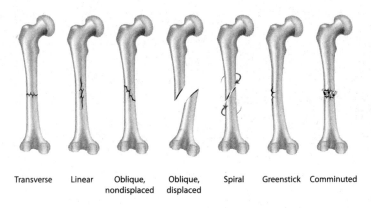

| Transverse | Linear | Oblique, nondisplaced | Oblique, displaced | Spiral | Greenstick | Comminuted |

Source: Orthopedic Institute at Southwest Health

Figure 17-1: Types of Bone Fractures

B. Strain

    1. A muscle or tendon injury due to over-stretching or tearing

    2. Causes pain and tenderness

    3. Usually little bleeding, swelling, or discoloration

C. Sprain

    1. Injury to a ligament, often involving the shoulder, knee, or ankle joints

    2. Signs and symptoms

        i.   Immediate pain and tenderness

        ii. Delayed swelling and bruising

D. Dislocation

    1. Movement of a bone out of its normal position in a joint.

    2. The bone may return to its normal position or remain out of joint.

3. Signs and symptoms

   i. Pain, deformity

   ii. Loss of function

   iii. Weak or absent distal pulses

Note: An orthopedic injury with absent distal pulses is a potentially limb-threatening injury. The patient should be regarded as a high transport priority.

E. Potential Limb-Threatening Injuries

1. Any orthopedic injury with loss of distal circulation is a high priority. The limb is at risk until circulation is restored.

2. Signs of orthopedic injury with poor distal circulation

   i. Absent distal pulses

   ii. Pallor distal to injury

   iii. Cold-to-touch distal to injury

   iv. Delayed capillary refill distal to injury

   v. Low SpO_2 distal to injury

F. Potential Life-Threatening Musculoskeletal Injuries

1. Pelvic fractures

   i. Pelvic fractures can cause life-threatening bleeding.

   ii. One out of five hip fracture patients die within one year of the injury.

   iii. Hip fracture patients are at risk for hypovolemic shock, pulmonary embolism, pneumonia, and sepsis.

   iv. Most hip fractures are due to fall injuries in elderly patients.

   v. Pelvic binders may help stabilize a pelvic fracture and reduce bleeding.

2. Femur fractures

   i. Femur fracture patients are at increased risk for hypovolemic shock, pulmonary embolism, pneumonia, and sepsis.

      ii.   Suspect other injuries if the patient has fractured the strongest bone in the body.

   3. Amputations

      i.   Control bleeding.

      ii.   Wrap amputated part in a sterile dressing, place in plastic, and keep cool.

      iii. Do **not** delay transport of patient to recover an amputated part.

      iv. Do **not** place an amputated part directly on ice.

III. SPLINTING

A. Splinting (when done correctly) can help decrease pain and reduce the risk of further injury.

B. Incorrect splinting

   1. Increases pain

   2. Reduces circulation to injured area

C. Rules of splinting

   1. Do **not** delay transport of a high-priority patient to splint a non-life-threatening injury.

   2. Assess distal pulse, motor function, and sensation (PMS) before and after splinting.

      i.   Pulse: Assess pulse distal to injury.

      ii.   Motor: Assess patient's ability to move the extremity distal to the injury.

      iii. Sensation: Assess patient's ability to sense touch distal to the injury.

      iv. Reassessment: PMS should be assessed regularly after the splint is applied. Assess for signs and symptoms that the splint is too tight.

   3. Immobilize above and below the injury.

      i.   Long-bone injuries: Immobilize the bone and the joints above and below the injury.

      ii.   Joint injuries: Immobilize the joint and the bones above and below.

   4. Attempt to realign deformed injuries **if** distal pulse is absent.

      i.   Make one attempt to realign with gentle, inline traction and reassess pulses (per local protocol).

      ii.   If distal pulse is not restored, treat as a high-priority patient.

      iii. If severe pain, crepitus, or resistance is encountered, stop and immobilize as is.

D. Types of splints include cardboard splints, padded board splints, wire splints, formable splints, pneumatic splints, vacuum splints, traction splints, pillow splints, and pelvic binders.

   1. Specialized splints

      i.   Traction splints: specifically for isolated, closed, midshaft femur fractures. Do **not** delay transport of a high-priority patient to apply a traction splint.

      ii.   Pelvic binder: consider for patients with a suspected pelvic fracture.

III. SPECIAL SITUATIONS

A. Suspected musculoskeletal injuries to the spine: Follow local protocol regarding spinal motion restriction.

B. Pediatric patients

   1. Musculoskeletal injuries to pediatric patients can permanently damage bone growth and function if not managed properly.

   2. Overuse injuries are common in youths aged 6 to 18 who participate in organized athletics.

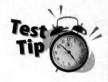

Test Tip

Complete as many (good) practice questions as you can before taking the certification exam. You should review at least 100 practice questions for each of the five categories on the exam, as well as pediatrics, CPR, and patient assessment. Use them to identify content you need to study further before the test.

PRACTICE QUESTIONS
Answers on page 388.

1. You should suspect a limb-threatening injury for any orthopedic injury with

   A. deformity.

   B. swelling.

   C. poor distal circulation.

   D. associated contusions.

2. What is the most common cause of hip fractures in elderly patients?

   A. fall injuries

   B. motor vehicle accidents

   C. pathologic fractures

   D. elder abuse

3. Which of the following fractures are most likely to cause life-threatening bleeding, pulmonary embolism, or sepsis? (Select the TWO answer options that apply.)

   A. radial fracture

   B. femur fracture

   C. tibial fracture

   D. clavicular fracture

   E. pelvic fracture

4. Which of the following is your highest priority for a patient with an amputation injury?

   A. Wrap the amputated part carefully before transport.

   B. Assure the patient that there will be no permanent damage.

   C. Control any significant bleeding.

   D. Rapidly place the amputated part on ice.

5. Your patient has a suspected fracture of the forearm. You should immobilize

   A. the humerus, elbow, and forearm.

   B. the elbow, forearm, and wrist.

   C. the forearm only.

   D. the humerus, elbow, forearm, and wrist.

Head and Spinal Injuries

I. TERMS TO KNOW

A. Anisocoria: Unequal pupils.

B. Anterograde amnesia: Inability to remember events that occurred after an injury.

C. Intracranial pressure: Pressure within the cranium.

D. Priapism: Persistent penile erection unrelated to sexual arousal.

E. Retrograde amnesia: Inability to remember events that occurred before an injury.

II. HEAD INJURIES

A. Pathophysiology

    1. Traumatic brain injury (TBI) accounts for about 30% of all trauma-related deaths.

    2. The risk of death doubles for TBI patients with hypotension or hypoxia.

B. Head injuries include trauma to the scalp, skull, and brain.

    1. Scalp injuries may indicate deeper, more serious head injury.

    2. Skull injuries indicate an even greater likelihood of brain injury.

C. Scalp

    1. Scalp injuries can be open or closed.

    2. The scalp is highly vascular and can bleed significantly.

D. Skull fractures

   1. Linear fractures

      i. The bone is fractured but does not move.

      ii. Most skull fractures are linear and do not present with deformity or depression.

   2. Depressed fractures

      i. Depression or deformity are more likely.

      ii. Increased risk of brain injury if bone is displaced into the brain.

   3. Basal skull fractures

      i. Fractures at the base of the skull

      ii. Cerebral spinal fluid (CSF) may leak from the nose or ears.

      iii. Signs may include:

         ➤ Battle's sign: bruising behind the ears (mastoid area)

         ➤ Raccoon eyes: bruising under the eyes

E. Brain injuries

   1. Concussion

      i. A concussion is a mild form of traumatic brain injury (TBI) that causes temporary dysfunction of the brain.

      ii. Signs and symptoms typically appear rapidly and gradually improve, including:

         ➤ Altered LOC (dazed, confused)

         ➤ Brief loss of consciousness

         ➤ Nausea and vomiting

         ➤ Headache

         ➤ Tired or lethargic

         ➤ Personality changes, irritability

         ➤ Repetitive questioning or answers questions slowly

         ➤ Balance or vision problems

         ➤ Light or noise sensitivity

         ➤ Numbness or tingling

➤ Complains of "not feeling right"

➤ Amnesia (before or after event)

— Retrograde amnesia: Can't remember what happened before the injury.

— Anterograde amnesia: Can't remember what happened after the injury.

Note: Concussion symptoms generally get better over time, not worse. If your patient is getting worse, you should assume a more urgent form of traumatic brain injury.

2. Cerebral contusion

   i.   A cerebral contusion is bruising of the brain.

   ii. Often accompanied by edema or concussion.

   iii. Signs and symptoms include signs of concussion *and* at least one of the following:

   ➤ Decreasing mental status

   ➤ Unresponsive

   ➤ Pupillary changes

   ➤ Abnormal vital signs

   ➤ Behavioral abnormalities

3. Epidural hematoma

   i.   Bleeding beneath the skull but above the dura mater (outermost meningeal layer).

   ii. Frequently involves significant arterial bleeding.

   iii. High risk of significant brain damage due to increased intracranial pressure.

   iv. Most patients with an epidural hematoma also have a skull fracture.

   v.   Signs and symptoms

   ➤ Sudden and brief loss of consciousness. Patients often wake up and experience progressive deterioration in consciousness.

   ➤ Headache

> Seizures

> Vomiting

> Hypertension

> Bradycardia

> Abnormal respirations (may be fast, slow, or irregular)

> Pupillary changes

> Posturing

— Decorticate "toward the core" posturing: Muscles are rigid, arms are flexed, fists are clenched, and legs are straight.

— Decerebrate posturing: Muscles are rigid, arms and legs are extended, toes are pointed down, and head/neck are arched backward.

4. Subdural hematoma

   i. Bleeding above the brain, beneath the dura mater but above the arachnoid (middle) meningeal layer.

   ii. Often caused by venous bleeding following a cerebral contusion.

   iii. Signs and symptoms

   > Vomiting

   > Decreased LOC

   > Pupillary changes

   > Hypertension

   > Headache

   > Respiratory changes

   > Seizures

5. Subarachnoid hemorrhage

   i. Bleeding within the subarachnoid space

   ii. Blood can enter CSF

   iii. Can be caused by trauma or ruptured aneurysm

    iv. Signs and symptoms

      ➤ Headache

      ➤ Stiff neck (nuchal rigidity)

      ➤ Decreased LOC

      ➤ Seizures

6. Intracerebral hemorrhage

    i. Bleeding within brain tissue

    ii. Patients likely to deteriorate rapidly

    iii. High mortality rate (about 40% during first 30 days)

> *Note:* The brain is in an enclosed space. There is little room to accommodate swelling or bleeding before brain damage occurs due to increased pressure.

7. Herniation syndrome

    i. The pressure within the skull is called intracranial pressure (ICP). Herniation syndrome occurs when the brain is compressed due to excessive ICP.

    ii. Severely increased ICP will force brain tissue toward the foramen magnum.

    iii. Signs of increased ICP

      ➤ Cushing's response: Hypertension with widened pulse pressure, bradycardia, abnormal respirations. Also known as "Cushing's triad" or "Cushing's reflex." Indicates TBI with increased ICP.

      ➤ Mortality rates are high for patients with severely increased ICP.

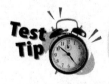

> Critical concept: You need to know what Cushing's response is and what it indicates before taking the certification exam.

8. Management of head injured patients

    i. There are three devastating things to avoid when caring for any patient with suspected traumatic brain injury (TBI).

➤ *No hypoxia.* Do not let the patient become hypoxic even once. Provide high-flow oxygen throughout care and transport. Hypoxia in a TBI patient can double the risk of death.

➤ *No hypotension:* Do your best to keep the patient from becoming hypotensive. Hypotension in a TBI patient can double the risk of death.

➤ *No hyperventilation.* Do **not** hyperventilate the patient with a BVM. This can decrease cerebral perfusion.

ii. Any patient with signs or symptoms of brain injury should be considered a high-transport priority.

iii. Treat for shock and transport rapidly to an appropriate facility per local protocol.

iv. Consider consulting medical control for any patient with signs of head injury who refuses transport (per local protocol).

III. SPINAL INJURIES

A. Mechanisms of Injury for Spinal Trauma

1. Flexion: extreme forward (chin to chest) movement of the head

2. Extension: extreme backward movement of the head, common in rear-impact collisions

3. Compression: compression of head against the body, such as a diving injury

4. Rotation: extreme lateral (side-to-side) movement

5. Distraction: stretching of the spinal column and cord, such as a hanging incident

6. Lateral bending: extreme bending of the head to the side (ear to shoulder)

7. Penetrating injury: open spinal injury, such as would result from a shooting or stabbing

B. Signs and Symptoms of Spinal Injury

1. The higher up the level of injury to the cervical spine, the more severe the symptoms are.

2. Pain, tenderness

3. Pulse, motor or sensory deficits

  i. **Pulse:** weak or absent radial or pedal pulses

  ii. **Motor:** weak or absent motor function (grip strength in hands and ability to push down or pull up with feet)

  iii. **Sensation:** ability to sense touch

4. Paralysis

  i. Paraplegia: paralysis of the lower extremities

  ii. Quadriplegia: paralysis of all four extremities

5. Priapism

C. Special Situations

1. Transected (severed) spinal cord

  i. Paralysis below the level of injury

  ii. Loss of bladder or bowel control

  iii. Respiratory paralysis (C1–C5 injury)

2. Neurogenic shock (see Chapter 15 for additional information)

  i. Hypotension without tachycardia

  ii. Possible respiratory paralysis

  iii. Priapism (uncontrolled penile erection)

  ➤ Priapism is associated with complete motor and sensory paraplegia.

  ➤ Does not always occur, but always occurs immediately with paraplegia.

3. Helmets

  i. In most cases, helmets can be left on during care and transport as long as the patient can be adequately assessed and managed.

  ii. If unable to adequately assess and manage the patient, the helmet should be removed with minimal movement of the cervical spine.

  iii. Follow local protocol regarding spinal motion restriction procedures.

4. Pediatric patients

    i. Pediatric patients have a large head in proportion to their bodies. This can cause hyperflexion of the head and spine while supine, complicating spinal motion restriction or airway/ventilation management.

    ii. Padding may be applied behind the shoulders to help keep the head and spine in a neutral, in-line position.

    iii. Do **not** use a car seat that has been involved in an accident during ambulance transport.

D. Management of Spinal Injuries

1. The end of "full spinal immobilization"

    i. The National Association of EMS Physicians, the American College of Emergency Physicians, the American College of Surgeons Committee on Trauma, and the National Registry of EMTs have all issued position statements calling for "spinal motion restriction" to replace "full spinal immobilization." This consensus, in most cases, has eliminated the use of the long spine board for immobilization in EMS.

    ii. Hazards of full spinal immobilization

       ➤ **Increased pain.** Healthy patients immobilized for just one hour report still being in pain 24 hours later.

       ➤ **Respiratory compromise.** Chest straps cause increased respiratory distress in all age groups.

       ➤ **Tissue damage.** Occipital tissue pressure and sacral tissue hypoxia develops in as little as 30 minutes.

       ➤ **Ineffective immobilization.** About 88% of patients in "full spinal immobilization" still had significant vertical and horizontal motion.

Note: The long spine board is now considered an extrication device. The patient should be removed from the long spine board as soon as possible.

2. The current standard is "spinal motion restriction."

    i. Indications

       ➤ Blunt trauma with altered LOC

       ➤ Spinal pain or tenderness

> ➤ Neurological compromise (numbness or weakness)

> ➤ Anatomic deformity of the spine

> ➤ High-energy mechanisms associated with intoxication, inability to communicate, or distracting injury

    ii.   Spinal motion restriction (SMR)

> ➤ Apply a rigid cervical collar.

> ➤ Carefully place patient on stretcher.

> ➤ Firmly strap patient in using stretcher seat belts.

> ➤ SMR does **not** include use of a long spine board.

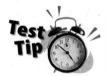

Review the National Registry's Resource Document on Spinal Motion Restriction/Immobilization prior to taking the national certification exam: *https://www.nremt.org/News/National-Registry-of-EMT-s-Resource-Document-on-Sp.*

PRACTICE QUESTIONS
Answers on page 389.

1. Battle's sign and raccoon eyes are indications of

    A. cervical spine injury.

    B. basal skull fracture.

    C. linear skull fracture.

    D. priapism.

2. Which of the following are used during spinal motion restriction? (Select the TWO answer options that apply.)

    A. long spine board

    B. rigid cervical collar

    C. ambulance stretcher

    D. head immobilizer

    E. medical duct tape

3. You are assessing a patient who was struck in the head by a softball. She is having difficulty remembering events prior to the injury. This is known as

   A. retrograde amnesia.

   B. anterograde amnesia.

   C. diffuse amnesia.

   D. concussive amnesia.

4. Your trauma patient presents with the following vitals: BP of 180/100, pulse of 56/minute, and respirations of 8/minute. You should suspect

   A. hypovolemic shock.

   B. neurogenic shock.

   C. TBI with increased ICP.

   D. concussion injury.

5. Your patient was struck in the head and immediately lost consciousness for a short time. The patient quickly woke up, but his mentation is now deteriorating. You should suspect

   A. a concussion.

   B. distraction injury to the spine.

   C. epidural hematoma.

   D. transient ischemic attack.

Chest and Abdominal Injuries

Note: See Chapters 15 and 16 for a review of internal bleeding and evisceration injury.

I. TERMS TO KNOW

A. **Hemothorax:** Accumulation of blood within the pleural space.

B. **Pericardial tamponade:** Accumulation of fluid in the pericardial sac.

C. **Simple pneumothorax:** Closed pulmonary injury where air leaks into the pleural space.

D. **Tension pneumothorax:** Pneumothorax causing progressive build-up of air in pleural space.

II. CHEST INJURIES

A. Pathophysiology

1. Second most common traumatic injury in non-intentional trauma.

2. Motor vehicle accidents are the most common cause of chest trauma.

3. Mortality is as high as 60%.

4. Chest injuries can be open or closed.

    5. Immediately life-threatening injuries:

       i. Significant hemothorax

       ii. Significant pneumothorax

       iii. Cardiac tamponade

    6. General signs and symptoms

       i. Pain, tenderness

       ii. Crepitus, paradoxical motion

       iii. Bruising and/or penetrating wounds

       iv. Dyspnea, hypoxia

       v. Hemoptysis

       vi. JVD (with obstructive shock)

       vii. Abnormal lung sounds (diminished or absent)

       viii. Hypotension, signs of shock

B. Types of Chest Injuries

    1. Pneumothorax

       i. Pneumothorax (simple pneumothorax) is the accumulation of air in the pleural space.

       ii. Lung tissue can be compressed/collapsed, leading to hypoxia.

       iii. Lung sounds may be diminished or absent over affected area.

    2. Tension pneumothorax

       i. A cause of obstructive shock.

       ii. Tension pneumothorax results when air is trapped in the pleural space under positive pressure. It can displace lung tissue, the mediastinum, and obstruct blood flow.

       iii. Signs and symptoms

          ➤ Severe respiratory distress, respiratory failure

          ➤ Diminished or absent lung sounds on affected side

          ➤ Tracheal deviation toward unaffected side (this is a **late** sign)

    3. Open pneumothorax ("sucking chest wound")

       i. Open chest wound with penetration into the pleural space.

    ii.   May allow air to enter pleural space during spontaneous inhalation.

    iii.   Penetrating wounds to chest or upper back should be covered with a vented occlusive dressing to prevent air from entering the chest cavity.

4. Hemothorax

    i.   Bleeding into the pleural space.

    ii.   Can lead to hypovolemic shock and respiratory compromise.

5. Cardiac tamponade ("pericardial tamponade")

    i.   A cause of obstructive shock.

    ii.   Occurs when blood or other fluid fills the pericardial sac and compresses the heart.

    iii.   The classic symptoms are "Beck's triad":

       ➤ JVD

       ➤ Muffled heart tones

       ➤ Narrowing pulse pressure / hypotension

> *Note:* Narrowing pulse pressure occurs when diastolic pressure rises and systolic pressure falls. Common causes include cardiac tamponade, tension pneumothorax, cardiogenic shock, severe hypovolemia.

6. Clavicle and rib fractures

    i.   Clavicle and rib fractures often indicate additional injuries, such as pneumothorax.

    ii.   Fractures to first several ribs indicate significant MOI.

    iii.   Signs and symptoms

       ➤ Pain & tenderness (especially on deep inspiration or palpation)

       ➤ Crepitus

      ➤ Subcutaneous emphysema (a "crackling" sensation upon palpation of the neck or chest)

7. Flail chest

    i.   Occurs when a portion of the ribcage becomes separated from the rest of the thorax.

    ii.   Caused by fracture of at least two consecutive ribs in two or more places.

    iii. Can also occur if sternum becomes separated from the ribcage.

    iv. Signs and symptoms

        ➤ Pain, tenderness to thorax

        ➤ Dyspnea

        ➤ Crepitus

        ➤ Possible paradoxical motion (when a portion of the chest wall appears to move in opposite direction from the rest of the thorax)

8. Traumatic aortic dissection

    i.   Traumatic rupture of aorta, usually due to blunt trauma from sudden deceleration.

    ii.   High fatality rate.

9. Traumatic asphyxia

    i.   Severe compression of the thorax that compromises blood flow.

    ii.   Causes a mechanical hypoxia due to external compression of chest.

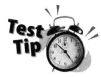

Patients with a suspected flail chest and inadequate breathing **must** be ventilated with a BVM. A bulky dressing, tape, sandbags, etc., are *not* the appropriate intervention for inadequate breathing.

III. ABDOMINAL INJURIES

A. Pathophysiology

    i.   Solid organs (spleen, liver, kidneys, pancreas) bleed when injured. The primary concern is hypovolemic shock.

    ii.   Hollow organs spill contents when ruptured. The primary concern is infection, such as peritonitis.

B. Signs and symptoms of abdominal injuries with possible internal bleeding

   i.   Pain, tenderness

   ii.   Distention, rigidity

   iii.   Bruising, guarding (stiffening of abdominal muscles)

   iv.   Kehr's sign (referred left shoulder pain on palpation of the abdomen while patient is supine with legs elevated)

   v.   Cullen's sign (umbilical bruising)

   vi.   Grey Turner's sign (bruising to left flank)

IV. SPECIAL PATIENTS

A. Elderly patients

   1.   Falls are the most common mechanism of injury for elderly patients.

   2.   Abdominal organs more prone to injury, especially the aorta, liver, and spleen.

B. Pediatric patients

   1.   Higher risk of car vs. pedestrian or car vs. bicycle accidents.

   2.   Chest and abdomen are not well protected.

   3.   Due to high pliability of the thorax, the absence of rib fractures does **not** rule out significant trauma.

C. Kidney injuries

   1.   Kidneys are well-protected, so kidney injuries are often accompanied by other injuries.

   2.   Signs and symptoms of possible kidney trauma

       i.   Flank pain

       ii.   Flank injuries (open or closed)

       iii.   Fractures to lower ribcage or lumbar region

       iv.   Hematuria

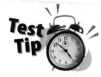

Here are a few critical concepts from this chapter. Get your flashcards ready!

1. What is the most important intervention for a flail chest with respiratory compromise?

2. What type of dressing should be applied to sucking chest wound?

3. What is Beck's triad and what does it indicate?

PRACTICE QUESTIONS
Answers on page 390.

1. Your patient has air trapped in the thorax under positive pressure. This is known as

   A. simple pneumothorax.

   B. hemothorax.

   C. pulmonary embolism.

   D. tension pneumothorax.

2. A sucking chest wound is also known as a(n)

   A. open pneumothorax.

   B. flail chest.

   C. hemothorax.

   D. pulmonary embolism.

3. Beck's triad includes which of the following? (Select the THREE answer options that apply.)

   A. JVD

   B. absent lung sounds

   C. muffled heart tones

   D. hypertension

   E. altered respirations

   F. narrowing pulse pressure

4. Your patient presents with paradoxical motion and severe respiratory distress. You should immediately do which of the following?

   A. Apply a bulky dressing to the chest.

   B. Administer oxygen via nasal cannula.

   C. Tape the patient's ribs.

   D. Begin BVM ventilations.

5. If your trauma patient presents with Kehr's sign, Cullen's sign, or Grey Turner's sign, you should suspect

   A. cardiac tamponade.

   B. internal bleeding.

   C. traumatic brain injury.

   D. kidney trauma.

Eye, Face, and Neck Injuries

I. TERMS TO KNOW

A. Conjunctiva: Membrane that covers the front of the eye and inside of the eyelids.

B. Cornea: Transparent, dome-shaped surface that covers the front of the eye.

C. Iris: Colored portion of the eye that surrounds the pupil.

D. Pupil: Round opening at the center of the iris.

E. Sclera: Visible white portion of the eye.

II. EYE INJURIES

A. Pathophysiology

   1. About 27% of serious eye injuries lead to legal blindness.

   2. Most common eye injuries

      i.   Corneal abrasion

      ii. Foreign objects in the eye

      iii. Chemical burns

      iv. Black eye due to blunt trauma

B. Corneal abrasion

   1. Both direct trauma and foreign objects can cause corneal abrasion.

      2. Symptoms

         i.   Pain

         ii. Tearing

         iii. Visual impairment

         iv. Sensation of something in the eye

C. Foreign Objects

      1. Non-penetrating foreign objects on the sclera can often be removed by irrigating the eye with sterile saline solution.

      2. Foreign objects in any other part of the eye and foreign objects on the sclera that are not removed by irrigation should be evaluated by a physician.

D. Chemical Burns

      1. Chemicals in the eyes should be immediately and continuously irrigated with sterile saline.

      2. Avoid irrigating chemicals from one eye into the other.

      3. A Morgan Lens is a device used for irrigating the eye. It resembles a contact lens connected to tubing. It is **not** typically used by EMTs.

Note: An IV bag of 0.9% sodium chloride ("normal saline") connected to blood tubing connected to a nasal cannula allows for continuous irrigation of the eyes. Place patient supine and place the nasal cannula on the bridge of the nose to irrigate medial to lateral (no chemical runoff from one eye to the other).

E. Blunt Trauma

      1. Blunt trauma can cause minor injuries such as a black eye, or more serious injury such as an orbital fracture.

      2. Orbital fracture

         i.   Orbital fractures indicate a significant mechanism of injury. Consider possibility of traumatic brain injury.

         ii. Signs and symptoms: visual disturbances, double vision, deformity around the orbit, inability to move eye in an upward gaze.

F. Conjunctivitis

1. A common eye infection, also known as pink eye.

2. Inflammation of the conjunctiva. Highly contagious.

3. Symptoms: redness, itching, tearing

G. Special Situations

1. Impaled objects

   i. Do **not** remove impaled objects from the eye.

   ii. Stabilize the object in place and keep both eyes closed/covered to prevent passive movement.

2. Contact lenses

   i. Contact lenses can usually be left in place; however, they may need to be removed in special situations (chemicals in the eyes).

   ii. Soft lenses can be easily removed by gently pulling down lower eyelid and pinching the lens. Hard contact lenses are best removed with a lens removal tool. Consult local protocol regarding removal of contact lenses.

3. Subconjunctival hemorrhage (broken blood vessels in the eye)

   i. Appears as redness to the sclera.

   ii. May be caused by coughing, sneezing.

   iii. Does **not** require treatment. Typically resolves within one or two weeks.

H. Assessment for increased intraocular pressure

1. Pupillary response normal or abnormal?

2. Loss of vision or vision acuity?

3. Halos, blurred or tunnel vision, blind spots?

4. Eye movement impaired?

5. Associated orbital or facial trauma?

6. Eye pain?

Note: Any eye injury with signs of increased intraocular pressure can lead to vision loss.

III. FACE INJURIES

A. Determine whether patient is on blood thinners (increased risk of hemorrhage, intracranial injury).

B. Dental Avulsion (loss of a tooth)

   1. Control bleeding and protect airway.

   2. Place tooth in saline-soaked gauze or whole milk.

C. Impaled Object in Cheek: Stabilize object in place unless it interferes with airway management or causes an airway obstruction.

D. Nosebleeds: See Chapter 15.

E. Ear injuries: Treat as soft tissue injury.

Note: Remember, bruising around the eyes or behind the ears may indicate serious head injury (basal skull fracture). See Chapter 18 for more information.

 IV. NECK INJURIES

A. Maintain high index of suspicion for underlying injuries from both blunt and penetrating neck trauma.

B. Primary concerns

   1. Massive hemorrhage

   2. Airway compromise

   3. Air embolism

C. Management

   1. Secure the airway.

   2. Control bleeding.

   3. Treat for shock as needed.

   4. Apply occlusive dressing to open neck wounds to reduce risk of air embolism.

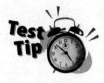

Use practice questions to help identify concepts or facts that need further study or memorization before the certification exam. Do not memorize the correct answers to specific questions; this is like memorizing the answer to a specific math problem instead of learning how to solve the problem.

PRACTICE QUESTIONS
Answers on page 390.

1. How should most cases of non-penetrating foreign objects on the sclera be managed?

   A. Bandage both eyes.

   B. Use a cotton swab to remove the object.

   C. Irrigate the eye with sterile saline or eye drops.

   D. Have the patient blink rapidly.

2. Your patient experienced blunt facial trauma. She complains of double vision, pain around her left eye, and is unable to gaze upward. You should suspect

   A. orbital fracture.

   B. corneal abrasion.

   C. mastoid fracture.

   D. maxillary trauma.

3. Your patient has a pencil impaled in one eye. Which of the following interventions are appropriate? (Select the TWO answer options that apply.)

   A. Remove the object.

   B. Apply gentle pressure to the pencil.

   C. Stabilize the pencil.

   D. Keep both eyes closed.

   E. Determine the range of motion for both eyes.

4. Your patient has experienced a traumatic dental avulsion. You should

    A. place the tooth in a biohazard bag.

    B. place the tooth in saline-soaked gauze.

    C. wrap the tooth in a dry, sterile dressing.

    D. place the tooth in skim milk.

5. What should be done to reduce the risk of air embolism for a large open neck wound?

    A. Apply a tourniquet.

    B. Apply an occlusive dressing.

    C. Place the patient prone with head down.

    D. Place gentle pressure on both sides of the neck.

Environmental Emergencies

I. TERMS TO KNOW

A. Barotrauma: Injury caused by a change in air pressure.

B. Frostbite: Cold emergency in which the tissue is frozen.

C. Hyperthermia: Systemic heat-related emergency.

D. Hypothermia: Systemic cold-related emergency.

E. Tinnitus: Ringing in the ears.

II. HEAT AND COLD EMERGENCIES

A. Factors Affecting Heat and Cold Emergencies

1. Age. The very young and very old do not tolerate heat and cold emergencies well.

2. General health. Those in poor health or poorly hydrated are more susceptible to heat and cold emergencies.

3. Environmental conditions. Extreme temperatures, humidity, and wind can all affect the body's ability to protect itself from heat and cold emergencies.

4. Medications and alcohol can both affect the body's ability to regulate body temperature.

B. Physiologic effects of heat and cold

1. Cold causes vasoconstriction (to conserve heat) and slowing metabolic rate.

2. Heat causes vasodilation (to shed excess heat) and increasing metabolic rate.

III. COLD EMERGENCIES

A. The Five Ways the Body Loses Heat

1. Conduction: Direct transfer of heat through contact with a colder structure. Example: bare feet on a cold floor.

2. Convection: Loss of heat to passing air. Example: being out in a cold breeze.

3. Evaporation: Loss of heat from being wet or sweating.

4. Respiration: The body warms and humidifies inhaled air, leading to loss of heat and body fluids.

5. Radiation: Transfer of radiant heat. Example: entering a walk-in freezer.

B. Hypothermia

1. Hypothermia is a systemic cold emergency that affects the entire body.

2. Hypothermia develops when the body's core temperature falls below what is needed to maintain homeostasis (below about 95° F (35° C).

3. Signs and symptoms

i. Signs and symptoms get worse as hypothermia progresses from mild, to moderate, to severe.

➤ Mild: 90–95° F (32°–35° C)

➤ Moderate: 82°–90° F (28–32° C)

➤ Severe: below 82° F (28° C)

ii. Skin

➤ Skin will be cold. Assess by feeling the torso, not the extremities or forehead.

➤ Follow local protocol regarding assessment of core temperature.

iii. Shivering

➤ Develops during mild hypothermia to increase body heat.

➤ Stops during moderate hypothermia.

iv. Coordination (muscle stiffness, difficulty speaking or moving)

v. Level of consciousness (LOC)

> ➤ LOC can range from confused (mild hypothermia) to comatose (severe hypothermia).

> ➤ Once patient reaches moderate hypothermia, they may wander into danger and even take off their clothes.

vi. Vitals

> ➤ Bradycardia, bradypnea, and hypotension develop as hypothermia worsens.

> ➤ Patients may appear to be in cardiac arrest even when they are not due to severe bradycardia and coma.

Note: Assessing mentation and level of consciousness are much faster assessments than core temperature. Patients with a decreased level of consciousness are in trouble.

4. Management of Hypothermia

i. Remove from the cold environment (ensure safety for yourself and your crew).

ii. Manage life-threatening conditions

> ➤ Unresponsive patients: check pulse for 30 to 45 seconds.

> ➤ Administer CPR as needed.

> ➤ Follow local protocol regarding AED use for hypothermic patients.

iii. Passive rewarming

> ➤ Remove wet clothing.

> ➤ Apply blankets.

> ➤ Turn heat on.

> ➤ Do **not** handle patient roughly, massage extremities, or rewarm too rapidly as these increase the risk of ventricular fibrillation.

C. Local Cold Emergencies

1. Local cold emergencies affect a specific part or parts of the body.

2. Hands, feet, nose, and ears are at highest risk for local cold injuries.

3. Frostnip

    i.   Mild frostbite with no permanent damage.

    ii.   Causes numbness to affected area with normal appearance.

    iii.   Pain or tingling is common as frostnip areas rewarm.

4. Trench foot

    i.   Also called immersion foot. Caused by prolonged exposure to water.

    ii.   Causes itching, pain, swelling, cold and blotchy skin, and possible blistering.

    iii.   Remove wet shoes and socks and allow to air dry.

5. Frostbite

    i.   The most dangerous local cold emergency.

    ii.   Tissue is frozen, often leading to permanent damage.

    iii.   Can cause gangrene (death of tissue), systemic infection, and death if not treated.

    iv.   Signs and symptoms

        ➤ Hard, frozen, waxy tissue.

        ➤ Possible blistering or mottling.

        ➤ Skin may be red, white, blue, gray, purple, brown, or ashen.

    v.   Management

        ➤ Remove from cold environment.

        ➤ Remove wet clothing.

        ➤ Protect affected areas from further injury.

        ➤ Remove any jewelry.

        ➤ Bandage and immobilize affected areas.

        ➤ Keep patient immobile.

        ➤ Do **not** massage affected areas.

        ➤ Do **not** apply direct heat unless directed by medical control.

IV. HEAT EMERGENCIES

A. Heat Cramps

1. Heat cramps are a local heat emergency.

2. Severe, involuntary muscle cramping that typically occurs during prolonged exertion.

3. Can affect legs or core muscles and is likely caused by dehydration and electrolyte imbalance.

4. Management includes rest, cool down, clear fluids with electrolytes, gentle stretching and massage.

B. Heat Exhaustion

1. Heat exhaustion is a common systemic heat emergency.

2. Caused by a combination of heat exposure (active or passive) and dehydration.

3. Signs and symptoms

   i. Exposure to warm environment

   ii. Dizziness, weakness

   iii. Nausea, vomiting

   iv. Headache, muscle cramps

   v. Tachycardia, thirst

   vi. Possible orthostatic hypotension

4. Management

   i. Remove from hot environment

   ii. Passive cooling

   iii. Rehydration

C. Heat Stroke

1. Uncommon and the most dangerous form of hyperthermia.

2. The body loses the ability to regulate body heat. Core temperature rises rapidly and will cause death if not managed rapidly.

3. Can develop due to active (working outside) or passive (child in a hot car) exposure to hot environment.

4. Signs and symptoms

    i. Similar to heat exhaustion

    ii. Altered or decreased LOC

    iii. Skin may be hot and dry or wet

    iv. Seizures

Note: During heat stroke, the patient will stop sweating. In a hot, dry environment, this will lead to hot, dry skin. In a hot, highly humid environment, the skin can stay wet even without active sweating.

5. Management

    i. Remove patient from hot environment.

    ii. Aggressive cooling measures

       ➤ Expose patient.

       ➤ Cold packs to groin, neck, armpits.

    iii. Rapid transport

    iv. Prepare for vomiting and/or seizures.

IV. DROWNING INCIDENTS

A. Pathophysiology of drowning incidents

1. Children ages 1 to 4 have the highest drowning rates.

2. After birth defects, drowning is the leading cause of death for children ages 1 to 4.

3. Second leading cause of injury-related deaths behind motor vehicle crashes for ages 1 to 14.

4. Hospital admission rate for drowning incidents is 5x higher than most other injuries.

5. Most pediatric drownings happen in swimming pools.

6. Almost 80% of drowning fatalities are male.

7. Two-thirds of infant drownings occur in bathtubs.

8. Arizona, California, Florida, and Texas have the most fatal pediatric drowning incidents.

9. Alcohol use, seizure history, failure to use PFDs (recreational water activities), and lapse of supervision are known risk factors for drowning incidents.

B. Do not attempt water rescue without proper training.

C. Drowning incidents pose several challenges for responders.

1. Potential respiratory and cardiac arrest

2. Potential trauma-related injuries

3. Potential hypothermia

4. Potential burn injuries (on concrete during summer months)

5. Chaotic scenes with distraught parents and bystanders

6. Emotionally difficult calls for many rescuers

D. Management

1. Manage respiratory and cardiac arrest as you normally would.

2. Treat as a high-priority trauma patient.

3. If the patient accepts an OPA, then ventilate with a BVM. Do **not** hyperventilate.

4. Have suction ready as vomiting is likely.

V. DIVING INJURIES

A. Descent Emergencies

1. Descent barotrauma ("the squeeze")

   i. Caused by lack of pressure equalization in closed spaces (ear, teeth, sinuses).

   ii. Signs and symptoms: ear pain, tinnitus (ringing in the ears), dizziness, hearing loss.

2. Nitrogen narcosis ("rapture of the deep")

   i. Drowsiness caused by breathing air under high atmospheric pressure.

   ii. Signs and symptoms: altered LOC, impaired judgment, intoxicated feeling.

B. Ascent Emergencies

1. Decompression sickness ("the bends")

   i. Caused by sudden decompression on ascent causing nitrogen bubbles to form in tissues.

   ii. Signs and symptoms: severe joint/abdominal pain, altered LOC, dizziness, nausea & vomiting, tinnitus, chest pain, cough, pulmonary edema.

   iii. *Note:* Flying too soon after a dive can cause decompression sickness.

2. Pulmonary overpressure

   i. Barotrauma usually due to held breath during ascent.

   ii. Can cause pneumothorax, arterial gas embolism, and air in the pericardial sac.

   iii. Signs and symptoms: chest pain, dyspnea, diminished breath sounds, signs of a stroke, narrowing pulse pressure.

C. General Management of Diving Emergencies

1. High-flow oxygen

2. Consider CPAP

3. Transport to hyperbaric chamber per local protocol

4. *Note:* Air medical transport may cause further harm due to altitude effects.

 VII. **HIGH ALTITUDE SICKNESS**

A. High altitude sickness is caused by exposure to high-altitude, low-oxygen environments.

B. Includes acute mountain sickness (AMS), high-altitude cerebral edema (HACE), and high-altitude pulmonary edema (HAPE).

C. Signs and symptoms: dizziness, weakness, dyspnea, altered LOC, chest pain.

D. Management

1. Halt ascent and descend as soon as possible.

2. High-flow oxygen.

3. Rapid transport.

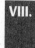 ## VIII. LIGHTNING INJURIES

A. High likelihood of respiratory and cardiac arrest.

B. Provide CPR and AED rapidly if cardiac arrest occurs.

C. Treat as a trauma patient.

 ## IX. BITES AND STINGS

A. General management of bites and stings

1. Move patient to safety if safe to do so.

2. Administer supportive care (thorough assessment, oxygen as needed, transport).

3. Assess for and manage systemic complications (such as shock, seizures) as needed.

4. Remove stingers.

5. Wash area.

6. Contact Poison Control or medical direction as needed.

B. Spiders

1. The brown recluse and black widow spiders both live in the United States and are potentially dangerous to humans.

2. Brown recluse

   i. Bites are not immediately painful and may not be noticed at the time.

   ii. Signs and symptoms

   ➤ Localized pain, redness, and swelling develop over several hours.

   ➤ Local tissue necrosis can develop over days to weeks.

   iii. Transport as needed.

2. Black widow

    i.   Bites to humans come from female black widow spiders.

    ii.   Signs and symptoms

       ➤ Immediate, localized pain, redness, and swelling

       ➤ Muscle spasms may develop

    iii. Transport as needed. *Note:* Antivenom is available for black widow envenomation.

C. Scorpions

1. Small children at higher risk of systemic complications from envenomation.

2. Signs and symptoms

    i.   Local pain, burning, numbness

    ii.   Slurred speech

    iii. Hyperactivity (especially in children)

    iv. Involuntary movement of the eyes (nystagmus)

    v.   Muscle twitching, excessive salivation

    vi. Abdominal cramps, nausea, and vomiting

    vii. Seizures

3. Management

    i.   Supportive care, have suction ready

    ii.   Transport

    iii. *Note:* Antivenom is available but poses significant risks

E. Snakebites

1. Do **not** . . .

    i.   apply ice, cold packs, etc.

    ii.   apply tourniquet.

    iii. cut wound.

    iv. attempt to suck the poison out.

    v.   apply electrical stimulation.

2. Signs and symptoms of poisonous snake bite

    i. Local pain, swelling, oozing at the wound site

    ii. Abdominal pain, nausea and vomiting, diarrhea

    iii. Dizziness, weakness, syncope

    iv. Shock or respiratory failure

    v. Seizures

    vi. *Note:* The onset of symptoms can be rapid or delayed for several hours.

3. General management of snakebites

    i. Wash wound site.

    ii. Immobilize bite site (follow local protocol regarding use of constricting bands or compression bandages).

    iii. Transport (consider antivenom availability).

F. Marine animals

1. Includes jellyfish, corals, stingrays, urchins

2. **All** can cause severe pain (heat typically reduces pain)

3. Signs and symptoms

    i. Intense local pain, nausea, and vomiting

    ii. Dyspnea, weakness, shock

4. Management

    i. Follow local protocol regarding use of constricting bands or compression bandages.

    ii. Apply heat (110°–113° F)

X. SPECIAL PATIENTS

A. Children left unattended in parked cars are at the greatest risk of heat stroke.

B. Infants, children, elderly, and obese persons are at the greatest risk of heat and cold related injury.

C. Alcohol consumption significantly increases the risk of drowning.

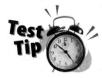

By now, you should have a growing list of information to memorize before the certification exam. Depending on your learning style, these may be in the form of notes, outlines, flashcards, etc. Commit to learning at least five new things each day. Be sure to include daily review of previously learned information each day. After a week, you will have memorized 35 things likely to be on the test. Most of them you will have reviewed multiple times (or soon will). This is the brain's version of sets and reps.

PRACTICE QUESTIONS
Answers on page 391.

1. Which of the following are common physiologic effects of cold exposure? (Select the TWO answer options that apply.)

   A. peripheral vasoconstriction

   B. peripheral vasodilation

   C. increased metabolic rate

   D. decreased metabolic rate

   E. fever

2. Which of the following are common physiologic effects of heat exposure? (Select the TWO answer options that apply.)

   A. peripheral vasoconstriction

   B. peripheral vasodilation

   C. increased metabolic rate

   D. decreased metabolic rate

   E. waxy skin

3. Rewarming a hypothermic patient too rapidly or rough handling can lead to

   A. ventricular fibrillation.

   B. combative behavior.

   C. hyperventilation syndrome.

   D. spinal injury.

4. Which of the following is a common systemic heat-related condition caused by heat exposure and dehydration?

A. heat stroke

B. local burns

C. heat exhaustion

D. trench foot

5. You suspect your patient is experiencing heat stroke. Your cooling measures must be

A. slow and cautious.

B. delayed until arrival at the hospital.

C. rapid and aggressive.

D. monitored with a rectal thermometer.

PART VI

MEDICAL, OBSTETRICS, AND GYNECOLOGY

REVIEW PLUS
END-OF-CHAPTER PRACTICE

Respiratory Emergencies

Note: A review of the respiratory section of Chapter 6 is recommended.

I. TERMS TO KNOW

A. **ARDS:** Acute respiratory distress syndrome.

B. **Dyspnea:** Difficulty breathing.

C. **Hemoptysis:** Coughing up blood.

D. **Orthopnea:** Difficulty breathing while lying down.

E. **RSV:** Respiratory syncytial virus.

II. PATHOPHYSIOLOGY

A. Chronic respiratory diseases, especially asthma and COPD, are a leading cause of illness and the sixth leading cause of death in the United States.

B. Respiratory emergencies can be caused by chronic or acute medical conditions or traumatic injuries.

C. Any patient complaining of respiratory distress should be transported for physician evaluation.

III. **RESPIRATORY DISTRESS/FAILURE/ARREST**

A. Respiratory distress (dyspnea): difficulty breathing. It can be mild, moderate, or severe.

1. Signs and symptoms

   i. Shortness of breath

   ii. Tachypnea

   iii. Abnormal lung sounds

   iv. Altered LOC (restless, anxious)

   v. Accessory muscle use

   vi. Cyanosis

   vii. SpO_2 below 94%

2. Examples of accessory muscle use

   i. Intercostal retractions

   ii. Abdominal breathing

   iii. Supraclavicular retractions

   iv. Tracheal tugging

   v. Sternal retractions

   vi. Nasal flaring

   vii. Tripod positional breathing

   viii. Seesaw breathing

   ix. Pursed-lip breathing

Note: **All** patients with respiratory distress should be placed on continuous SpO_2 monitoring.

3. General management

   i. Oxygen as needed to maintain SpO_2 of at least 94%

   ii. CPAP as indicated

   iii. Bronchodilators (albuterol, Atrovent) as indicated via MDI or SVN

   iv. Supportive care and transport

B. Respiratory failure: inadequate spontaneous breathing

    1. Signs and symptoms

        i.   Severe respiratory distress

        ii. Decreased LOC

        iii. Shallow breathing

        iv. Excessively fast or slow breathing

        v. Abnormal lung sounds

        vi. Difficulty speaking

        vii. Severe accessory muscle use

    2. Management

        i.   BVM ventilation connected to high-flow oxygen

        ii. No hyperventilation!

C. Respiratory arrest: no breathing (apnea)

        i.   Patients in respiratory arrest require BVM ventilation connected to high-flow oxygen (no hyperventilation).

        ii. Remember, patients in respiratory arrest may or may not have a pulse.

Note: The treatment for respiratory failure and respiratory arrest is the same: BVM ventilation; however, the patient presentations are very different.

 ## IV. CAUSES OF RESPIRATORY EMERGENCIES

A. Acute respiratory distress syndrome (ARDS)

    1. Non-cardiogenic pulmonary edema. Causes include sepsis, toxic inhalation, pneumonia, COVID-19.

    2. Typically follows a major illness or injury in already hospitalized patients.

B. Airway obstruction (see Chapter 10)

C. Anaphylaxis (see Chapter 15)

D. Asthma

    1. Chronic respiratory condition caused by bronchoconstriction and excess mucus production.

    2. Can be minor to acutely life-threatening.

    3. Common triggers include pollution, allergens, stress, exercise, respiratory infection.

    4. Signs and symptoms

        i. Wheezing (primarily on exhalation)

        ii. Absent lung sounds in severe cases

        iii. Coughing

E. Chronic obstructive pulmonary disease (COPD)

    1. Slow, chronic disease that obstructs and damages the alveoli.

    2. Includes chronic bronchitis and emphysema.

    3. Largely due to cigarette smoke.

    4. Signs and symptoms

        i. History of smoking or exposure to cigarette smoke

        ii. Chronic productive cough

        iii. Diminished lung sounds with prolonged expiratory phase

        iv. Wheezing

        v. "Barrel chest" appearance

        vi. COPD patients are often on home oxygen

Note: Avoid tunnel vision. There are many causes of respiratory distress that involve other body systems, such as cardiac problems, infection, trauma, etc.

F. Congestive heart failure

    1. CHF is a common cause of dyspnea.

    2. See Chapter 12 for more information.

G. Croup

    1. Also known as laryngotracheobronchitis. Inflammation of the pharynx, larynx, and trachea.

2. Highly infectious (airborne). Children from 6 months to 3 years at highest risk.

3. Signs and symptoms

    i.   Usually preceded by a cold and typically in the wintertime

    ii.   "Barking" cough

    iii. Stridor

H. Cystic fibrosis (CF)

1. Genetic disorder leading to thick mucus production and chronic lung infections.

2. Often causes death by early adulthood.

3. Signs and symptoms

    i.   Asthma-like symptoms

    ii.   Cough

    iii. Gastrointestinal problems

    iv. Poor weight gain

I. Flail chest (see Chapter 19)

J. Hyperventilation syndrome

1. Characterized by rapid breathing.

2. Often associated with distraught patients; however, it can be a sign of serious medical problem, such as pulmonary embolism.

3. Do **not** have a patient experiencing hyperventilation breathe into a paper bag or otherwise limit adequate oxygenation.

K. Inhalation injury: see Chapter 16.

L. Pneumonia

1. Pneumonia is an infection of the lungs. It is often a secondary infection (following flu, RSV, COVID-19).

2. Pneumonia is the leading cause of death due to infectious disease in children.

3. Any patient who aspirates is at high risk of developing pneumonia. About 30% of patients with aspiration pneumonia will die.

Note: Do **not** hyperventilate with the BVM! Hyperventilation leads to gastric distention and vomiting. Vomiting leads to aspiration. Aspiration leads to pneumonia. Pneumonia leads to death.

    4. Signs and symptoms

       i.   Fever

       ii. Dyspnea

       iii. Weakness

       iv. Productive cough

       v. History of recent illness, chronic illness, or terminal illness

M. Pneumothorax

    1. The accumulation of air in the pleural space. Can occur spontaneously or as a result of trauma (see Chapter 19).

    2. Asthma patients are at an increased risk of spontaneous pneumothorax.

    3. Patients being ventilated with a BVM are at increased risk of pneumothorax due to hyperventilation and over-pressurization.

    4. Signs and symptoms include dyspnea and diminished or absent lung sounds in the affected area.

N. Pulmonary edema

    1. The accumulation of fluid in the lungs.

    2. Causes include CHF, toxic inhalation, disease, and trauma.

    3. Signs and symptoms

       i.   Abnormal lung sounds (rales or crackles)

       ii. History of cardiac problems (previous MI, CHF)

       iii. Possible pedal edema (swelling of the feet, ankles)

       iv. Orthopnea (difficulty breathing while lying down)

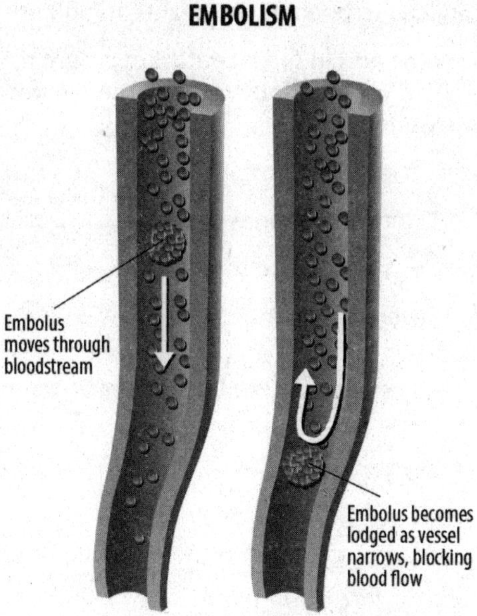

EMBOLISM

Embolus moves through bloodstream

Embolus becomes lodged as vessel narrows, blocking blood flow

Figure 22-1

O. Pulmonary embolism (PE)

1. The blockage of a pulmonary artery, usually a blood clot.

2. Risk factors for PE include recent surgery, long-bone fracture, deep vein thrombosis (DVT), being bedridden, stroke, hypertension, smoking, sitting for long periods, pregnancy, obesity, hormone therapy, birth control pills.

3. Signs and symptoms

   i.   Chest pain

   ii. Dyspnea, tachypnea

   iii. Hemoptysis

P. Respiratory syncytial virus (RSV)

1. A highly contagious respiratory infection common in infants and children.

2. Most children have contracted RSV by age 2.

3. Older adults are also at high risk for severe disease caused by RSV.

4. Can lead to pneumonia. Infants at high risk of severe complications.

5. Airborne and indirect contact exposure risk. RSV can live for hours on hard objects. Touching a contaminated object will most likely cause infection.

6. Signs and symptoms

   i. Congestion, runny nose

   ii. Dry cough, sore throat

   iii. Fever, headache

Q. Sucking chest wound and other thoracic trauma: see Chapter 19.

V. SPECIAL PATIENTS

A. RSV is the most common cause of pneumonia in pediatric patients.

B. Elderly patients and those recovering from surgery are at high risk of pneumonia.

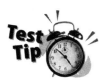

Test Tip

You must minimize interruptions in chest compressions for cardiac arrest patients. Compression fraction is the amount of time during resuscitation when compressions are being delivered. You must maintain 80+% compression fraction.

PRACTICE QUESTIONS
Answers on page 392.

1. Which of the following is a slow, chronic disease process that obstructs and damages the alveoli?

   A. asthma

   B. foreign body airway obstruction

   C. laryngotracheobronchitis

   D. COPD

2. You are caring for a 56-year-old patient with chest pain, dyspnea, tachypnea, and hemoptysis. You should suspect

   A. a pulmonary embolism.

   B. respiratory syncytial virus.

   C. cystic fibrosis.

   D. a stroke.

3. Which of the following are correct regarding respiratory syncytial virus (RSV)? (Select the TWO answer options that apply.)

   A. Elderly patients are at the highest risk of RSV.

   B. The RSV virus only lives for a few seconds on hard surfaces.

   C. RSV is a bloodborne pathogen.

   D. Most children have contracted RSV by age two.

   E. RSV causes a dry nose and a wet cough.

4. Which of the following is characterized by rapid breathing and is often associated with distraught patients?

   A. COPD

   B. RSV

   C. Hyperventilation syndrome

   D. Laryngotracheobronchitis

5. Select the appropriate management of a patient with respiratory distress. (Select the THREE answer options that apply.)

   A. Use continuous SpO_2 monitoring.

   B. Hyperventilate with a BVM.

   C. Use CPAP as indicated.

   D. Have patient breathe into a paper bag.

   E. Administer oxygen to maintain an SpO_2 of at least 90%.

   F. Consider albuterol or Atrovent MDI or SVN.

Endocrine and Hematologic Emergencies

I. TERMS TO KNOW

A. DKA: Diabetic ketoacidosis.

B. Kussmaul respirations: Deep, rapid respirations due to metabolic acidosis.

C. Polydipsia: Excessive thirst.

D. Polyphagia: Excessive hunger.

E. Polyuria: Excessive urination.

II. METABOLISM AND ENERGY PRODUCTION

A. Energy Sources

    1. Glucose

    2. Fat

    3. Protein

B. Glucose

    1. Glucose is the body's primary and preferred fuel source.

    2. Glucose is the only fuel source used by the brain.

    3. The brain must have a continuous supply of glucose.

    4. Glucose metabolism is an aerobic (with adequate oxygen) process. It is efficient and creates safe byproducts (water and CO_2).

C. Fats and Proteins

   1. The body can use these alternate fuel sources, but the brain cannot.

   2. Fat and protein metabolism is an anaerobic (without adequate oxygen) process. It is less efficient and creates dangerous by-products (lactic acid).

III. INSULIN AND BLOOD GLUCOSE

A. When glucose enters the body, it quickly enters the bloodstream (about 15 minutes).

B. Insulin (a pancreatic hormone) is needed to efficiently move glucose from the bloodstream into the cells for energy.

C. Insulin causes blood glucose levels to drop as the glucose enters the bloodstream.

D. An absence of insulin causes glucose to remain in the bloodstream and blood glucose levels will rise.

E. While most of the body can use alternate fuel sources (fat, protein), the brain must have glucose.

F. While most of the body's cells require insulin to receive glucose, the brain can receive glucose with or without insulin. This means:

   i.   The brain will be in trouble quickly if there is no glucose.

   ii.   The brain will be able to receive glucose if present regardless of the presence of insulin.

IV. TESTING BLOOD GLUCOSE LEVELS

A. A glucometer is used to assess blood glucose levels by testing a small drop of blood in just a few seconds.

B. In the United States, glucometers measure blood glucose levels in milligrams per deciliter (mg/dL). Some countries, such as Canada, assess blood glucose levels by molecular weight (mmol/L).

C. Blood glucose numbers

1. Fasting results: Ideally, blood glucose levels are tested after fasting. A fasting blood glucose level of 99 mg/dL or less is normal. A fasting blood glucose level of 100 mg/dL or higher indicates possible prediabetes or diabetes.

2. Non-fasting results: For EMS purposes, a "normal" blood glucose level is 80 to 120 mg/dL. *Note:* A blood glucose level of 140 mg/dL just after eating is not unusual.

   i. Hyperglycemia: a blood glucose level above normal

   ii. Hypoglycemia: a blood glucose level below normal

D. Continuous glucose monitoring and automated insulin delivery is now possible for diabetics using an insulin pump with a tiny sensor placed under the skin (usually on the abdomen or arm). The sensor tests glucose levels every few minutes and transmits the data to a monitor, phone, etc.

E. A1C blood glucose testing averages blood sugar levels over several months. The results are reported as a percentage. A normal A1C level is below 5.7%. Above 5.7% indicates chronic hyperglycemia.

V. DIABETES

A. Pathophysiology of diabetes

1. Diabetes is a disease caused by inadequate insulin production in the pancreas and/or insulin resistance.

2. Untreated diabetes typically causes hyperglycemia.

3. Once the blood glucose level reaches about 200 mg/dL, glucose begins to spill into the urine for elimination. The increased urinary output can lead to dehydration, hypovolemia, and shock.

B. Type 1 diabetes

1. Also called insulin-dependent diabetes. Type 1 diabetic patients create little or no insulin and must take supplemental insulin.

2. Type 1 diabetes usually develops by young adulthood. Only 5%–10% of diabetics are type 1. There is a strong genetic component to type 1 diabetes.

3. The Three P's: Untreated type 1 diabetes will typically present with . . .

    i.   Polydipsia: excessive thirst (due to increased urinary output)

    ii. Polyphagia: excessive hunger (the body wants glucose)

    iii. Polyuria: excessive urination (due to hyperglycemia)

4. Type 1 diabetics are at risk of developing diabetic ketoacidosis (DKA). This is a life-threatening emergency caused by excessively high blood glucose levels (over about 300 mg/dL).

5. Type 1 diabetics are at risk of insulin shock (aka "diabetic shock") caused by an insulin overdose. Insulin shock is a life-threatening emergency caused by severe hypoglycemia (below 70 mg/dL).

C. Type 2 diabetes

1. Also called non-insulin dependent diabetes. Type 2 diabetics do not typically require insulin, but it may be necessary as the disease progresses and diet, exercise, and other medications cease to be effective.

2. Obesity and genetics are common causes. About 90%–95% of diabetics have type 2 diabetes.

D. Complications of diabetes

1. Fatty deposits in blood vessels increase the risk of heart attack and stroke.

2. Chronic hyperglycemia damages the circulatory system and can lead to blindness and amputation of the lower extremities due to ulcers that won't heal.

VI.   SPECIFIC DIABETIC EMERGENCIES

A. Insulin shock

1. Insulin shock ("diabetic shock") is a severe, symptomatic form of hypoglycemia.

2. Insulin shock can develop rapidly and is a life-threatening emergency that can rapidly lead to brain damage.

3. Causes

    i.   Insulin overdose

    ii. Regular insulin dose and not eating

      iii. Extreme physical activity without adjusting insulin dose and food intake

    4. Signs and symptoms

      i. Low blood sugar

      ii. Acute onset confusion, irritability, abnormal behavior

      iii. Diaphoresis, pale/cool/clammy skin

      iv. Tachycardia

      iv. Coma

      v. Seizures

Note: Glucagon is a potentially life-saving medication for severe hypoglycemia. It can be administered intramuscularly or intranasally. This can prevent severe brain damage or death in an unresponsive diabetic in insulin shock who cannot be given oral glucose. There is no identifiable reason why EMTs everywhere are not authorized to carry and administer glucagon.

  B. Diabetic ketoacidosis (DKA)

    1. DKA is severe hyperglycemia (over 300 mg/dL) caused by a lack of insulin.

    2. The brain can receive glucose without insulin; however, the rest of the body will switch to a backup fuel source. This leads to anaerobic metabolism and acidosis.

    3. Signs and symptoms

      i. Hyperglycemia (typically over 300 mg/dL)

      ii. Kussmaul (deep, rapid) respirations due to acidosis

      iii. Flushed, hot, dry skin

      iv. Coma, often with urinary incontinence

      v. Seizures

      vi. Excessive hunger, thirst, and urination (The Three P's)

      vii. Fruity or acetone odor on breath

  C. Hyperglycemic hyperosmolar nonketotic syndrome (HHNS)

    1. Similar to DKA, but typically occurs with type 2 diabetes

    2. Very slow onset (days to weeks)

3. Often caused by an infection, poor management of blood glucose levels, or failure to take diabetic medication as prescribed

D. Management of suspected diabetic emergency

1. Scene safety, as always, is the first priority.

2. Manage immediate life threats (coma, seizures, shock, etc.).

3. Administer oxygen.

4. Assess blood glucose level.

5. Follow local protocols regarding medication administration (such as oral glucose) and ALS response.

6. Transport.

Note: Remember, hypoglycemic patients **must** have a secure airway and the ability to swallow to receive oral glucose.

VII. HEMATOLOGIC EMERGENCIES

A. Hematologic disorders involve the blood and/or blood-forming organs (bone marrow, lymph nodes, spleen).

B. Hemophilia

1. Clotting disorder causing poor bleeding control. Almost always occurs in males.

2. Signs and symptoms include extensive bruising and bleeding that is difficult to control.

3. Hemophilia patients often have a medical alert bracelet.

4. Management includes bleeding control (compression, elevation), treatment for shock, and rapid transport.

C. Sickle cell disease

1. A form of inherited, chronic anemia.

2. In the U.S., African Americans are disproportionately affected by sickle cell disease.

3. Causes misshapen, rigid, and sticky red blood cells that do not carry oxygen efficiently and die prematurely.

4. Blood "sludges" and obstructs microvasculature, increasing risk of renal failure, stroke, and sepsis.

5. Signs and symptoms

    i.   Muscle and abdominal pain

    ii. Swelling of hands, feet

    iii. Frequent infections

6. Management includes oxygen administration and transport.

D. Leukemia

1. Cancer of the body's blood-forming tissues. White males over age 65 at highest risk.

2. Signs and symptoms include weakness, fever, weight loss.

VIII. SPECIAL PATIENTS

A. Rates of type 1 and type 2 diabetes are increasing in children.

B. Obesity is a significant risk factor for type 2 diabetes in all age groups. About one-third of children in the U.S. are overweight and about 40% of adults are obese.

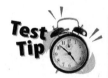

Test Tip

Severe hyperglycemia (DKA) typically takes at least several hours to develop and must be corrected in the hospital.

Severe hypoglycemia (insulin shock) can develop in minutes and requires aggressive intervention to get the blood sugar back up.

Both DKA and insulin shock can lead to seizure, coma, and death. The difference is insulin shock develops much faster and requires immediate action to raise the blood sugar.

PRACTICE QUESTIONS
Answers on page 392.

1. Insulin will cause blood glucose levels to

   A. decrease.

   B. increase.

   C. be unpredictable.

   D. fluctuate wildly.

2. Which of the following are the Three P's of untreated Type 1 diabetes? (Select the THREE answer options that apply.)

   A. polydactyly

   B. poliomyelitis

   C. polydipsia

   D. polyphagia

   E. polyuria

   F. polysaccharide

3. Which of the following is a normal, non-fasting blood glucose level?

   A. 40–60 mg/dL

   B. 70–120 mg/dL

   C. 120–160 mg/dL

   D. 160–200 mg/dL

4. If a person's blood glucose level exceeds 300 mg/dL, which of the following is most likely?

   A. acute hypertension

   B. pale, cool, clammy skin

   C. slow, shallow breathing

   D. increased urinary output

5. Which of the following interventions is recommended for a patient experiencing a sickle cell crisis?

A. oxygen

B. oral glucose

C. tourniquet application

D. obtain a signed refusal

Anaphylaxis and Toxicology

 I. **TERMS TO KNOW**

A. **Anaphylaxis:** Life-threatening allergic reaction, aka anaphylactic shock.

B. **Antibodies:** Proteins produced by immune system to attack antigens.

C. **Antigens:** Substances that produce an immune response.

D. **Epinephrine:** Medication used to treat anaphylaxis.

E. **Immunoglobulin E (IgE):** Antibodies that trigger an anaphylactic response ("IgE mediated anaphylaxis").

II. **ANAPHYLAXIS**

A. Pathophysiology of Anaphylaxis

1. Antigens are foreign substances that enter the body.

2. When antigens enter the body, they can trigger an immune response.

3. Antigens can be absorbed, ingested, injected, or inhaled.

4. Antibodies are produced by the immune system to attack antigens.

5. In most cases, anaphylaxis is caused by antibodies called immunoglobulin E (IgE).

B. Allergic Reaction

1. An allergic reaction is an excessive immune response to an allergen.

2. Allergic reactions can be local or systemic. Symptoms often include itchy skin, watery eyes, runny nose, rash, etc.

3. Sensitization

   i. Patients can develop sensitivity to a substance that did not previously cause a reaction.

   ii. Following sensitization, the severity of reactions can get progressively worse.

C. Anaphylactic Shock ("Anaphylaxis")

1. A severe, life-threatening form of allergic reaction

2. A form of distributive shock (see Chapter 15 for additional information)

3. Anaphylaxis is a severe, systemic allergic reaction, that can compromise the airway, respiratory, and cardiovascular systems.

4. Anaphylaxis is usually caused by the presence of antibodies called immunoglobulin E (IgE).

5. Signs and symptoms

   i. Airway swelling, hives

   ii. Stridor, wheezing, pulmonary edema

   iii. Hypotension, tachycardia

   iv. Increased mucus production

Note: At least three things are threatening your anaphylactic patient's life: airway swelling, bronchoconstriction, and hypotension.

D. Causes of Anaphylaxis

1. The most common causes of anaphylaxis are food (nuts, shellfish, eggs, etc.), medications (antibiotics, aspirin, etc.), and insect bites/stings (bees, wasps).

2. Latex and environmental triggers can also cause anaphylaxis.

E. Management: anaphylaxis patients require aggressive intervention

1. Secure the airway, give oxygen, and ventilate as needed.

2. Treat for shock.

3. Administer epinephrine auto-injector per local protocol.

4. Rapid transport.

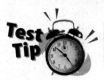 It is essential to understand the impact of vasodilation and bronchoconstriction on anaphylaxis. Bronchoconstriction causes severe respiratory distress and hypotension causes shock. Epinephrine administration can help with both.

III. TOXICOLOGY

A. Pathophysiology of Toxicology

1. Accidental poisonings are more common in pediatric patients but are less often fatal.

2. Poisonings in adults are less frequent but more often fatal.

3. Toxins can enter the body through ingestion, inhalation, injection, and absorption. Ingestion is the most common.

4. 90% of poisonings occur in the home. Almost half of poisonings occur in children under age 6.

Note: You can contact Poison Control 24/7 for information by calling 1-800-222-1222 (U.S. only).

B. Ingested Toxins

1. The most common route of exposure

2. An overdose of cardiac medications, psychiatric medications, opioids, or acetaminophen is extremely dangerous.

3. Intentional overdoses by adults frequently involve more than one substance.

4. Signs and symptoms

    i. Abdominal pain, cramps, nausea, and vomiting

      ii. Altered LOC, seizures

      iii. Burns to mouth and airway with strong acids and alkalis

   5. Consider activated charcoal per local protocol.

C. Inhalation

   1. Often involves chemicals, pesticides, carbon monoxide, or natural gas.

   2. Ensure scene safety, especially when there are multiple patients.

   3. Signs and symptoms: dyspnea, cough, headache, altered LOC.

D. Injection

   1. Most injected toxins are due to drug abuse. Onset of effects is usually rapid.

   2. Be alert for needles.

   3. Injection of stimulants (cocaine, amphetamines) will cause excitability and tachycardia. Can cause seizures, heart attack, stroke, and death.

   4. Injection of depressants, such as opioids, will cause respiratory depression and decreased LOC. Can cause seizures or coma, respiratory arrest, and death. Most opioids cause pupillary constriction.

E. Absorption

   1. Often involves pesticides and various acids/alkalis, or petroleum-based products.

   2. Signs and symptoms acids/alkalis, petroleum-based products: burns to skin, rash or blisters.

   3. Signs and symptoms of pesticide exposure: SLUDGEM or DUMBELS.

   4. The patient should be decontaminated as appropriate before transport. Most chemicals should be irrigated continuously with water for at least 20 minutes.

   5. Some chemicals react violently to water. Consult the Emergency Response Guidebook, fire department personnel, medical direction, or Poison Control for guidance.

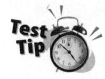

 You *must* know the signs and symptoms of exposure to pesticides and nerve agents. Use the SLUDGEM or DUMBELS acronym.

Salivation	**D**efecation
Lacrimation (tearing)	**U**rination
Urination	**M**uscle weakness
Defecation	**B**radycardia/Bronchospasm
Gastric upset (abdominal cramps)	**E**mesis
Emesis (vomiting)	**L**acrimation
Miosis (pupillary constriction)	**S**alivation

IV. TOXIDROMES

A. Toxidromes are a common collection of signs and symptoms associated with different classes of poisons. For example, you don't need to know the name of every opioid to know that all opioids cause similar signs and symptoms during an overdose.

B. Alcohol

1. There are several types of alcohol. Only ethanol is intended for consumption.

2. Alcohol abuse is common. Most long-term alcoholics develop serious health issues, such as hepatitis.

3. Alcohol is a CNS depressant and increases the risk of vomiting.

4. Alcohol withdrawal (delirium tremens) can be extremely dangerous.

C. Opioids

1. Opioids can be ingested, injected, or inhaled.

2. Examples: morphine, codeine, oxycodone, hydrocodone, heroin, fentanyl, and many others.

3. Opioids cause CNS depression and respiratory depression. In severe cases they cause coma, respiratory arrest, and death.

4. Most opioids cause significant pupillary constriction ("pinpoint pupils").

5. Administer naloxone for suspected opioid overdose per local protocol.

D. Sedative Hypnotics

1. CNS depressants that cause a calming, hypnotic effect, and sleep.

2. Examples: benzodiazepine and barbiturate medications, such as Valium, Xanax, amobarbital, secobarbital.

3. Usually ingested. Have been used to facilitate sexual assault.

E. Inhalants

1. Abused inhalants may include acetones, glues, cleaning chemicals, paints, aerosols, and propellants.

2. Can cause severe brain damage and cardiac arrest.

3. Signs of abuse include chemical odor on breath, paint stains on hands/clothes, apathy, weight loss.

4. Prescription and over-the-counter inhalers are also widely abused for stimulant effects or perceived advantage in competitive sports.

F. Stimulants

1. Stimulants include nicotine, caffeine, cocaine, amphetamines, "bath salts," guarana, taurine, and L-carnitine.

2. Signs and symptoms include dilated pupils, restlessness, anxiousness, agitation, paranoia, hallucinations, and excited delirium.

3. Can be taken by any route. Large doses can cause violent behavior, paranoia, anxiety, panic, seizures, headache, chest pain, and sudden cardiac arrest.

G. Hallucinogens

1. Hallucinogens alter sensory perception.

2. Can cause tachycardia, tachypnea, insomnia, diaphoresis.

3. Examples include LSD, psilocybin mushrooms (aka "magic mushrooms"), and PCP.

H. Acids and Alkalis

1. Acids and alkalis are both caustic substances. Found in many household products.

2. Acids burn on contact and usually cause immediate pain.

3. Alkalis tend to burn deeper. The onset of pain may be delayed.

4. Most caustic ingestions involve children.

5. Activated charcoal is **not** indicated in cases of ingested acids and alkalis.

I. Hydrocarbons

1. Hydrocarbons are petroleum-based. Found in gasoline, paints, solvents, sunscreen, and more.

2. Most hydrocarbon ingestion patients are children.

3. Contact Poison Control or medical direction for assistance.

4. Activated charcoal is **not** indicated for hydrocarbon ingestion.

V. SPECIAL PATIENTS

A. Pediatric patients

1. Batteries: swallowing batteries is extremely dangerous. Batteries can burn through a child's esophagus in only 2 hours. Lithium coin batteries are most hazardous.

2. Magnets: ingestion of magnets can lead to severe intestinal damage, hemorrhage, and death.

3. e-cigarettes: liquid nicotine is dangerous when swallowed.

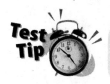

Always administer oxygen, check blood glucose levels, and consider naloxone for any patient with an altered or decreased LOC.

B. Drug abuse

1. Tolerance: Diminished response to a drug is due to repeated use.

2. Dependence: The body needs the drug.

3. Addiction: Addiction is defined by behavior. Tolerance and dependence lead to addiction. Substance abuse will continue despite negative consequences.

C. Carbon Monoxide (CO)

1. CO poisoning is a leading cause of death due to fires. Other common sources include home heating devices and vehicle exhaust.

2. CO inhibits the body's ability to transport and use oxygen.

3. CO is a silent killer. It is tasteless, colorless, odorless, and completely non-irritating when inhaled. Victims are usually unaware they are being exposed and become unconscious.

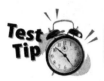 **Test Tip** Remember, the national certification exam does not let you go back and change your answer to previous questions. Read carefully before making your selection.

PRACTICE QUESTIONS
Answers on page 393.

1. Anaphylaxis causes which of the following? (Select the THREE answer options that apply.)

   A. bronchoconstriction

   B. bronchodilation

   C. vasoconstriction

   D. vasodilation

   E. hypotension

   F. hypertension

2. Administration of an epinephrine auto-injector is indicated for

   A. any patient experiencing an allergic reaction.

   B. patients with signs and symptoms of anaphylaxis.

   C. patients with sneezing, runny nose, and watery eyes.

   D. any patient with signs of an opioid overdose.

3. An overdose on sedatives or opioids is most likely to cause

   A. excitation.

   B. tachycardia.

   C. CNS depression.

   D. hypertension.

4. Your patient is unresponsive, breathing slow and shallow, and has pinpoint pupils. You should suspect

   A. amphetamine overdose.

   B. a pesticide exposure.

   C. inhalant abuse.

   D. opioid overdose.

5. Bath salts and methamphetamine are

   A. stimulants.

   B. depressants.

   C. opioids.

   D. cannabis.

Obstetrics and Newborns

 I. TERMS TO KNOW

A. Bloody show: Passage of a mucus plug from the vagina during the first stage of labor.

B. Gravida: Total number of pregnancies a woman has had, including a current pregnancy.

C. Para: Total number of pregnancies past 20 weeks in duration.

D. Postpartum: After childbirth.

E. Supine hypotensive syndrome: Caused by compression of the inferior vena cava when a pregnant patient is supine.

 II. GESTATIONAL DEVELOPMENT

A. A full-term pregnancy is 40 weeks.

B. Pregnancy is divided into three 13-week trimesters.

  1. First trimester: The embryo grows from fertilized egg into a moving fetus, with eyes, ears, and functioning organs.

  2. Second trimester: Features develop and the mother will likely begin to feel movement.

  3. Third trimester: The fetus grows rapidly during the final stage.

III. ANATOMICAL AND PHYSIOLOGICAL CHANGES IN PREGNANCY

A. Reproductive changes in mom

1. Uterine blood flow during pregnancy is 20x greater than prior to pregnancy.

2. The enlarging uterus displaces other internal structures.

B. Respiratory changes in mom

1. Respiratory rate increases slightly; however, oxygen demand increases significantly.

2. In the late stage of pregnancy, the diaphragm is frequently compressed by the enlarging uterus.

Note: The pregnant patient is at risk of developing hypoxia rapidly. Monitor breathing status and SpO_2 carefully. When in doubt, administer oxygen.

C. Cardiovascular changes in mom

1. Cardiac workload increases significantly.

2. Resting heart rate and blood volume increase.

3. Plasma increase is greater than red blood cells, leading to relative anemia.

4. Signs and symptoms of shock can be masked during pregnancy.

5. Supine hypotensive syndrome (from mom laying supine) can crash blood pressure.

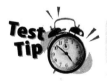

Test Tip

Do *not* allow the pregnant patient to lay supine. This can cause supine hypotensive syndrome and crash her BP. Tilt mom to her left side to avoid compressing the inferior vena cava.

D. GI and GU changes in mom

1. The pregnant patient likely has undigested food in her stomach, increasing the risk of vomiting and aspiration.

2. Pregnancy increases urinary frequency and increases the risk of bladder injury during trauma.

E. Musculoskeletal changes in mom

1. The center of gravity changes, increasing the risk of fall injury.

2. Hip, knee, and foot pain as well as leg spasms are common during pregnancy.

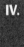 **IV.** **PATIENT HISTORY**

A. Are you pregnant? How many weeks? Due date?

B. Are you having contractions? Has your water broken?

C. How many pregnancies have you had (gravida)? How many deliveries have you had (para)?

D. Are you receiving prenatal care? Any known complications?

E. Are you expecting twins?

F. Any abdominal pain or vaginal bleeding?

G. Any recent trauma, including falls?

Note: Remember to provide emotional support to your pregnant patient. Depending on the reason for calling you, she may be experiencing extreme stress.

V. **LABOR AND DELIVERY**

A. Stages of labor

1. First stage

   i. Begins with the onset of contractions and ends with full cervical dilation.

   ii. The cervix is fully dilated at 10 cm, allowing infant's head to enter the birth canal.

   iii. Contractions initially occur at widespread intervals and become more severe and closer together over time.

   iv. The mucus plug (and some blood) that seals the uterine opening passes, aka "bloody show."

   v. The amniotic sac may rupture spontaneously.

   vi. Stage one typically lasts longer for first-time pregnancies.

2. Second stage

   i. Begins with full cervical dilation and ends with delivery of the baby.

   ii. Contractions are close together.

   iii. Mother feels intense pressure and urge to push.

3. Third stage

   i. Begins once baby is delivered and ends with delivery of the placenta.

   ii. Placenta typically delivers within 30 minutes after delivery of the baby.

   iii. There will be an increase in vaginal bleeding shortly before the placenta delivers and the mother will feel the urge to push again.

B. Transport or deliver on scene

1. Transport the mother to the hospital for delivery whenever possible. If delivery appears imminent, you should prepare to deliver on scene.

2. Consult medical direction to assist with decision.

3. The following are indications of possible imminent delivery:

    i.   The mother has strong, frequent contractions under 2 minutes apart with little break between contractions. *Note:* Contractions are timed from the beginning of one contraction to the beginning of the next contraction.

    ii. The abdomen is rigid during contractions.

    iii. The mother feels the urge to push.

    iv. Mother may report passage of mucus plug and/or rupture of the amniotic sac.

    v.   Crowning

        ➤ Crowning is the appearance of the baby's head in the birth canal.

        ➤ Assess for crowning if you suspect imminent delivery.

C. Preparing for delivery

1. Prepare OB kit.

2. Position the mother: not supine! Semi-reclined, knees drawn, bottom slightly elevated, feet planted.

3. Expose vaginal opening, assess for crowning, and apply clean sheets around birth area.

4. Tear the amniotic sac if it has not already ruptured.

5. Apply gentle pressure to neonate's skull (avoid fontanelles) as head presents in birth canal.

6. As the neonate's head delivers, check if the cord is wrapped around the neck (nuchal cord). If the cord is around the neonate's neck, gently remove it from around the neck. Be extremely cautious about clamping and cutting the cord, especially if multiple births is a possibility.

7. Suctioning the neonate

    i.   Routine suction of the neonate's mouth and nose is **not** recommended.

    ii. Suction fluid from the neonate's mouth and nose **only** if they are full of secretions **and** they do not start breathing on their own after drying and rubbing their back.

iii. Neonates born through meconium-stained amniotic fluid who do **not** start breathing on their own should be suctioned before initiating positive pressure ventilation.

8. Guide the presenting shoulder gently up. Once it clears, gently guide the baby downward to help clear the other shoulder. Never pull on the baby.

9. Support the baby upon delivery.

10. Begin assessment and management of the newborn.

11. Clamp and cut the cord once it stops pulsating.

12. Prepare for delivery of the placenta. Gently guide placental delivery, but never pull.

13. Uterine massage and breastfeeding can help reduce postpartum hemorrhage.

14. Transport mother, baby, and placenta.

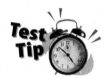

 Be sure you know the three key assessments for newborns: respirations, heart rate, and skin color. Getting the newborn's heart rate above 100 and keeping it there are essential.

VI. NEWBORN (NEONATAL) CARE

A. Immediately upon delivery, place on clean, dry sheets or towels.

B. Dry baby, including the head and immediately replace wet linen with dry.

C. Warm the baby, including the head. Placing the baby on the mother's abdomen will provide a radiant heat source.

D. If the baby is not active and crying, attempt tactile stimulation by rubbing the baby's back, or tapping the soles of the feet.

E. Assess respirations

1. If the baby is not breathing adequately, begin ventilations (40–60 per minute) with an appropriately sized bag and mask for 30 seconds with high flow oxygen.

2. Do **not** overinflate the newborn's chest (stop when chest rises).

F. Assess heart rate

1. Heart rate below 60 per minute: begin chest compressions and ventilations at 3:1 ratio.

2. Heart rate above 60 but below 100: provide ventilations.

3. Heart rate above 100: assess skin color.

G. Assess skin color: if central cyanosis is present, provide blow-by oxygen at about 4–6 lpm with oxygen tubing near the baby's face until color improved.

H. APGAR score

CRITERIA	0	1	2
Appearance	Cyanotic	Cyanotic extremities	No cyanosis
Pulse	Under 60	60–100	Over 100
Grimace	No response	Grimace or feeble cry when stimulated	Cries or pulls away when stimulated
Activity	Absent/limp	Some movement	Active movement
Respirations	Absent	Gasping, weak	Strong cry

 VII. TRAUMA IN PREGNANCY

Note: One in eight women are abused during pregnancy. The risk of homicide is 35% higher in women who are pregnant or postpartum.

A. Pregnant patients are at an increased risk of injury and death due to:

1. Motor vehicle accidents

2. Fall injuries

3. Domestic violence

B. Any injury to the mother can pose significant risk to the fetus.

   1. The physiological changes that occur during pregnancy mask the usual signs and symptoms of shock.

   2. Maintain an extremely high index of suspicion for any pregnant patient who experiences trauma, even in the absence of obvious signs and symptoms of injury, shock, or hypoxia.

   3. The fetus may be in serious jeopardy even if the mother appears uninjured.

C. Management of the pregnant trauma patient

   1. Conduct a thorough assessment.

   2. Determine specifics about the pregnancy while gathering the SAMPLE history.

   3. Do **not** place the pregnant patient supine due to the risk of supine hypotensive syndrome.

   4. Administer high-flow oxygen.

   5. Transport to an appropriate facility. If unsure, request ALS or contact medical direction.

 VIII. **OBSTETRICAL EMERGENCIES**

A. Hemorrhage

   1. Hemorrhagic shock can develop quickly in the pregnant patient.

   2. Signs and symptoms may not be evident until the pregnant patient is in severe shock.

   3. Bleeding can occur with little or no external blood loss.

   4. Bleeding may be painful or painless.

   5. Several conditions can lead to severe bleeding, including placenta previa, abruptio placenta, ectopic pregnancy, uterine rupture, spontaneous abortion.

B. Placenta previa

1. A common cause of bleeding in the third trimester.

2. Placenta previa occurs when the placenta attaches to the uterus over the cervical opening.

3. As the cervix dilates, the placenta is torn and bleeds.

4. Classic presentation is painless vaginal bleeding in the third trimester.

5. Assess for signs and symptoms of shock.

C. Abruptio placenta

1. Abruptio placenta is the premature separation of the placenta from the uterine wall, leading to bleeding.

2. Oxygen and nutrient delivery to fetus is compromised.

3. Maternal blood loss can be severe.

4. The fetus will not survive a complete abruption.

5. Classic presentation is painful vaginal bleeding in the third trimester.

6. Assess for signs and symptoms of shock.

D. Ectopic pregnancy

1. Ectopic pregnancy occurs when the egg is implanted outside of the uterus, usually in the fallopian tube.

2. Ectopic pregnancy can lead to rupture and severe bleeding.

3. Classic presentation is severe abdominal pain with or without vaginal bleeding.

4. Assess for signs and symptoms of shock.

E. Uterine rupture

1. The uterus thins as it grows, increasing the risk of rupture.

2. Danger to mother and fetus is high.

3. Classic presentation is abdominal pain and vaginal bleeding.

F. Spontaneous abortion

1. Spontaneous abortion (miscarriage) is delivery of the fetus before it is capable of surviving. This is prior to about the 20th–22nd week of pregnancy.

2. Classic presentation includes cramping in the lower abdominal pain, vaginal bleeding, and passage of tissue or clots.

3. Assess for signs and symptoms of shock.

G. Seizures

1. Pregnancy can increase the risk of seizures in the mother.

2. Management of seizures during pregnancy

i. Treat as regular seizures (see Chapter 13).

ii. Place patient on left side.

iii. Minimize exposure to stimulus such as lights, noise, and movement.

H. Preeclampsia and eclampsia

1. Preeclampsia (toxemia of pregnancy) typically occurs in the third trimester.

i. Cause is not completely understood.

ii. Signs and symptoms include sudden weight gain, visual disturbances, sudden swelling of the face, hands, feet, headache and hypertension.

2. Eclampsia

i. Eclampsia occurs when the mother seizes following preeclampsia.

ii. Eclampsia is a life-threatening condition for mother and fetus.

I. Pregnancy-induced hypertension (PIH)

i. PIH can develop in pregnant women after about 20 weeks gestation.

ii. PIH is defined as a blood pressure greater than 140 systolic and greater than 90 diastolic on at least two occasions at least 6 hours apart.

iii. PIH can also present with the same signs and symptoms as preeclampsia.

J. Supine hypotensive syndrome

i. Supine hypotensive syndrome occurs when the fetus compresses the inferior vena cava. This can cause a severe drop in blood pressure.

ii. Typically occurs in the later stages of pregnancy when the mother is supine.

iii. Signs and symptoms include dizziness, hypotension, pale skin, and altered level of consciousness.

iv. Management of supine hypotensive syndrome must include keeping the fetus off the inferior vena cava.

v. Do **not** place the patient in a supine position. Place the patient in a seated position or on her left side.

IX. DELIVERY COMPLICATIONS

A. Meconium

1. Meconium is the presence of fetal stool in the amniotic fluid. This turns the amniotic fluid yellow, green, or brownish.

2. The risk of infection and pneumonia increases if the baby inhales meconium.

3. If meconium is present, suction the mouth and nose promptly when the head clears the birth canal.

4. Once the baby delivers, immediately suction the mouth and nose prior to stimulating the baby to breathe.

B. Multiple births

1. Multiple births can have their own placenta, or share a placenta.

2. Be prepared for multiple births anytime it has not been ruled out by ultrasound.

3. Request additional units.

4. Prepare additional supplies, OB kits, BVMs, oxygen tanks, etc.

5. Be prepared for possible breech presentation, particularly with second baby.

6. Multiple birth babies may be smaller and require additional resuscitation efforts.

7. Clamp and cut an umbilical cord with possible multiple births only as a last resort.

8. If second baby does not deliver within about 10 minutes after first, transport immediately.

C. Prolapsed cord

1. A prolapsed cord occurs when the cord is the presenting part in the birth canal.

2. Prolapsed cord can become compressed and cut off oxygen to the baby.

3. Instruct the mother not to push. This will increase pressure on the cord.

4. Place mother in knee–chest position.

5. Carefully push the presenting part of the baby away from the cord.

6. Transport immediately.

D. Breech presentation

1. A breech birth occurs when the baby's buttocks or legs are the first presenting part in the birth canal.

2. Transport immediately. Breech births present significant dangers for mother and baby.

3. If delivery occurs, there is a high risk the head will become stuck in the birth canal.

4. If the head is trapped, use fingers to form a "V" along the vaginal wall to create space allowing the baby to breathe.

E. Limb presentation

1. A limb presentation is when a single arm or leg is the first presenting part in the birth canal.

2. Do **not** attempt delivery of a limb presentation in the field.

3. Place the mother in the knee–chest position and transport immediately.

F. Postpartum hemorrhage

    1. Postpartum hemorrhage is excessive bleeding following delivery.

    2. Blood loss of greater than about 500 mL is considered abnormal.

    3. Management of postpartum hemorrhage includes uterine massage, breastfeeding, and treating for shock.

G. Pulmonary embolism (PE)

    1. PE during pregnancy is not common; however, it accounts for 1 in 10 maternal deaths. Most of these deaths occur after delivery.

    2. Signs and symptoms: acute dyspnea, chest pain, sudden cardiac arrest.

H. Maternal cardiac arrest

    1. Begin CPR per current AHA BLS guidelines.

    2. Provide continuous lateral uterine displacement for pregnant patients in cardiac arrest.

    3. Do **not** use mechanical CPR devices on maternal cardiac arrest patients.

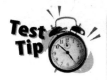

Test Tip

Most of the questions on the exam call for only one correct answer. You will often identify two answer choices that sound correct. Reread the question carefully. There will be something in the question to point you to the better answer choice.

PRACTICE QUESTIONS
Answers on page 394.

1. Which of the following statements regarding changes during pregnancy are correct? (Select the TWO answer options that apply.)

   A. The mother's cardiac workload decreases.

   B. Pregnant women are prone to anemia.

   C. Signs of shock are more obvious in pregnant patients.

   D. Pregnant patients should be placed supine during transport.

   E. Hypertension in pregnant patients is cause for concern.

2. Your patient is experiencing abdominal pain and vaginal bleeding during her third trimester of pregnancy. Which of the following is most likely?

   A. abruptio placenta

   B. preeclampsia

   C. pregnancy-induced hypertension

   D. supine hypotensive syndrome

3. Your patient is 37 weeks pregnant. She is complaining of headache, blurred vision, and swelling. You should suspect

   A. preeclampsia.

   B. eclampsia.

   C. ectopic pregnancy.

   D. uterine rupture.

4. Your patient has just delivered a full-term newborn. The newborn's heart rate is 70. You should

   A. begin chest compressions.

   B. deliver blow-by oxygen.

   C. initiate transport.

   D. provide bag-valve-mask ventilations.

5. Your patient is 35 weeks pregnant. You find her supine in bed complaining of weakness and nausea. You should be immediately concerned about

   A. hypertensive crisis.

   B. gestational diabetes.

   C. supine hypotensive syndrome.

   D. domestic abuse.

Abdominal and Gynecological Emergencies

Note: Many patients with abdominal pain will require surgery. It can be extremely difficult to determine the specific cause of a patient's abdominal pain. Do **not** delay care or transport of the patient to attempt a diagnosis. Treat the patient's presenting signs and symptoms, assess and manage shock as needed, and transport.

I. TERMS TO KNOW

A. **Hematemesis:** Vomiting blood.

B. **Hematochezia:** Bloody stool.

C. **Melena:** Dark, tarry stool.

D. **Peritonitis:** Inflammation of the peritoneum.

E. **Referred pain:** Pain felt somewhere other than where it originates.

II. ACUTE ABDOMINAL PAIN

A. Pathophysiology

1. The most common non-traumatic causes of acute abdominal pain are gastritis, appendicitis, gallbladder problems, UTI, kidney problems, peritonitis, and bowel obstruction.

2. Just over half of patients with acute abdominal pain are discharged from the ED.

3. Just over 25% of patients with acute abdominal pain require surgery.

B. Types of abdominal pain

  1. Acute onset: rapid, unexpected

  2. Visceral pain

    i. Dull, diffuse, difficult to localize

    ii. Frequently associated with nausea and vomiting

  3. Parietal

    i. Severe and localized. Usually sharp and constant

    ii. Patient often curls up with knees to chest

  4. Referred pain: Pain in an area of the body other than the source

C. Common signs and symptoms of abdominal emergencies

  1. Severe abdominal pain

  2. Kehr's sign (referred pain to left shoulder upon palpation of the abdomen)

  3. Hematemesis (vomiting blood)

  4. Hematochezia (bloody stool)

  5. Melena (dark, tarry stool)

  6. "Coffee-ground" appearing emesis (vomiting partially digested blood)

  7. Cullen's sign (bruising around the umbilicus)

  8. Grey Turner's sign (flank bruising)

  9. Abdominal guarding, rigidity or distention

  10. Signs and symptoms of shock

D. Causes of acute abdominal pain

  1. Gastroenteritis

    i. Intestinal infection causing cramps, diarrhea, vomiting, fever

    ii. May be contagious, depending on the cause (contaminated food or water, norovirus)

    iii. Can lead to hypovolemic shock, especially in children

  2. Appendicitis

    i. Inflammation of the appendix.

    ii.   If untreated, can lead to life-threatening infection (peritonitis) and septic shock.

    iii. Usually occurs in teens or 20s, but can occur at any age.

    iv. Signs and symptoms

- Abdominal pain that often starts as diffuse and periumbilical, then localizes to right lower quadrant.
- Increased pain with coughing, walking, jarring movements
- Nausea & vomiting
- Diarrhea, loss of appetite
- Fever

3. Peritonitis

    i.   Inflammation of the peritoneum, often due to a hole in the bowel or ruptured appendix.

    ii. Signs and symptoms: nausea & vomiting, loss of appetite, diarrhea, fever.

    iii. Surgery and antibiotics are required.

4. Cholecystitis

    i.   Inflammation of the gallbladder, often due to gallstones.

    ii. Risk factors: female, over age 40, obesity, diabetes, family history.

    iii. Signs and symptoms

- Right upper quadrant pain
- Increased pain at night and after eating fatty foods
- Referred shoulder pain
- Nausea and vomiting

5. Bowel obstruction

    i.   Occurs when food or stool cannot move through the intestines.

    ii. Can cause bowel necrosis and life-threatening infection (peritonitis).

    iii. Signs and symptoms: severe abdominal pain, nausea & vomiting, inability to pass gas or stool. May vomit stool.

6. Diverticulitis

   i. Inflammation or infection in the small pouches of the digestive tract.

   ii. Typically affects people over age 40 with a low-fiber diet.

   iii. Signs and symptoms: abdominal pain (usually left lower quadrant), fever, nausea, and vomiting.

7. Gastrointestinal bleeding

   i. Non-traumatic GI bleeding usually occurs in middle-aged or elderly patients.

   ii. High fatality risk in geriatric patients.

   iii. Upper GI bleeds often due to ulcers. Lower GI bleeds often due to diverticulitis.

   iv. Signs and symptoms

      ➤ Hematemesis

      ➤ Hematochezia

      ➤ Melena

      ➤ "Coffee-ground" appearing emesis

      ➤ Abdominal rigidity or distention

      ➤ Signs and symptoms of shock

8. Esophageal varices

   i. Enlarged veins in the esophagus.

   ii. Often seen in patients with advanced liver disease, such as alcoholics.

   iii. If ruptured, can lead to severe bleeding and shock.

   iv. Signs and symptoms: vomiting bright red blood.

9. Ulcers

   i. Open wounds along the digestive tract, often the stomach.

   ii. Signs and symptoms: abdominal pain, nausea and vomiting, increased pain before meals and during stress.

10. Hepatitis

   i. Inflammation of the liver.

   ii. Often associated with alcohol abuse.

   iii. High fatality rate for hepatitis B.

   iv. Can be spread by exposure to infected body fluids.

   v. Signs and symptoms: jaundice (yellow) skin, yellow sclera (whites of the eyes), right upper quadrant abdominal tenderness, loss of appetite, nausea & vomiting.

11. Aortic aneurysm

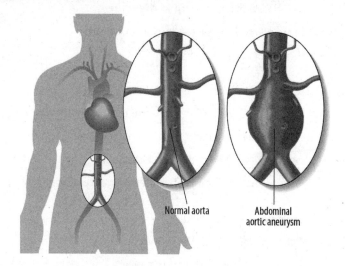

Normal aorta   Abdominal aortic aneurysm

   i. A weakening of the wall of the aorta.

   ii. Typically, they develop along the abdominal aorta (abdominal aortic aneurysm, or AAA) or along the thoracic region of the aorta.

   iii. The weakened area of aorta is prone to rupture. Rupture of an AAA will likely cause rapid, fatal hemorrhage.

   iv. Most often occurs in elderly males.

   v. Signs and symptoms

     ➤ "Tearing" back pain

     ➤ Possible pulsating abdominal mass

     ➤ Significant difference in blood pressures between left and right arms

III. GENITOURINARY CONDITIONS

A. Acute renal failure

    1. A sudden and dangerous (but potentially reversible) drop in urinary output.

    2. Kidneys are suddenly unable to filter waste products from the blood and excrete them in the urine.

    3. Most often occurs in seriously ill or injured patients.

    4. High mortality rate.

B. Chronic renal failure

    1. Inadequate kidney function due to irreversible kidney damage.

    2. Often caused by diabetes or hypertension.

    3. Typically requires dialysis or kidney transplant.

    4. Risks of dialysis include hypotension, infection, and hemorrhage.

C. Kidney stones (renal calculi)

    1. Calcium deposits in the kidneys.

    2. Signs and symptoms include severe flank pain, nausea & vomiting, hematuria, painful urination.

D. Urinary tract infection (UTI)

    1. Most common in females, paraplegics, and sexually active persons.

    2. Signs and symptoms: painful and frequent urination, foul smelling urine, history of UTIs, fever, back/flank/lower abdominal pain.

IV. GYNECOLOGICAL EMERGENCIES

A. Ectopic pregnancy

    1. Pregnancy where the fertilized egg implants outside of the uterus, usually in the fallopian tubes.

    2. A ruptured fallopian tube will cause massive hemorrhage that requires surgical intervention.

3. Signs and symptoms

   i.   Diffuse abdominal tenderness progressing to sharp, localized, unilateral lower quadrant abdominal pain.

   ii. The pain may radiate to the shoulder.

   iii. Late or missed menstrual cycle.

   iv. Vaginal bleeding.

   v.   Signs and symptoms of shock.

Note: Any sexually active female between the onset of menstruation and menopause with abdominal pain should be evaluated for ectopic pregnancy.

B. Pelvic inflammatory disease (PID)

   1. Infection of the female reproductive tract, including gonorrhea and chlamydia.

   2. Can be acute or chronic.

   3. If untreated, PID can lead to infertility, ectopic pregnancy, sepsis, and cancer.

   4. Signs and symptoms

      i.   Diffuse lower abdominal pain

      ii. Increased pain with intercourse or walking

      iii. Fever and chills

      iv. Nausea and vomiting

      v.   Foul-smelling vaginal discharge

      vi. Mid-cycle vaginal bleeding

C. Sexual assault

   1. Victims of sexual assault can be male, female, or non-binary.

   2. The first priority is patient care, then reporting to the appropriate authorities.

   3. Guidelines for management of sexual assault victims

      i.   Treat the patient first. Preserve evidence second.

      ii. Provide emotional support.

   iii. Provide same-sex EMS provider when possible.

   iv. Do not disrupt the scene any more than necessary to treat the patient.

   v. Handle clothing as little as possible.

   vi. Place any clothing or bloody items that have been removed in brown paper bags, not plastic bags.

   vii. Do not cut through tears or holes in clothing.

   viii. Examine the genitalia only if necessary.

   ix. Encourage the patient not to change clothes, urinate, shower, or douche prior to medical examination at the hospital.

   x. Treat the patient's injuries as needed and transport.

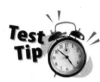

Consider creating "pathophysiology" flashcards for common medical emergencies and traumatic injuries. Include common signs and symptoms for each condition. These can be extremely helpful when trying to determine the most likely cause of the patient's condition.

Sample Patho Card (front): "Describe the pathophysiology of hypovolemic shock, and the common signs and symptoms."

Sample Patho Card (back): "Hypovolemic shock is inadequate tissue perfusion due to fluid loss. It usually presents with tachycardia, restlessness, and pale/cool/clammy skin."

PRACTICE QUESTIONS
Answers on page 394.

1. Your patient complains of acute abdominal pain. This means the pain

   A. is severe.

   B. is sharp.

   C. started suddenly.

   D. requires surgery.

2. Which of the following symptoms most likely indicate internal abdominal bleeding? (Select the THREE answer options that apply.)

A. vomiting blood

B. coffee-ground emesis

C. fever

D. painful urination

E. nausea

F. melena

3. Your patient complains of abdominal pain that is dull, diffuse, and difficult to localize. This is known as

A. visceral pain.

B. acute pain.

C. parietal pain.

D. referred pain.

4. Your 17-year-old patient is complaining of abdominal pain. He states it was "all over" but now is localized to his right lower quadrant. The patient denies any trauma and has never had any surgeries. Which of the following is most likely?

A. cholecystitis

B. diverticulitis

C. acute renal failure

D. appendicitis

5. Which of the following is an intestinal infection associated with nausea, vomiting, and diarrhea?

A. gonorrhea

B. pancreatitis

C. renal calculi

D. gastroenteritis

Behavioral Emergencies

I. TERMS TO KNOW

A. **Agitated delirium:** Delirium characterized by agitation, aggression, acute distress, aka "excited delirium."

B. **Behavioral emergency:** A situation where a person's behavior presents an imminent risk of serious harm or death to self or others.

C. **Delirium:** Acute onset of cognitive problems.

D. **Dementia:** Slow onset of memory impairment.

E. **Dysarthria:** Difficulty speaking.

II. PATHOPHYSIOLOGY OF BEHAVIORAL DISORDERS

A. Physiological causes include diabetic emergency, hypoxia, head injury, drugs, alcohol, toxins, infection, etc.

B. Psychological causes include

1. anxiety: an unusual level of stress.

2. bipolar disorder: unusual shifts in mood, energy, concentration. Formerly known as manic depression.

3. depression: deep sadness not associated with a specific event.

4. paranoia: extreme suspicion or distrust of others without justification.

5. phobias: extreme fear of something specific.

6. psychosis: delusional state where contact with external reality is lost.

7. schizophrenia: disorganized thoughts, perceptions, emotions, and social interactions.

C. Social causes include bullying, abuse, family conflict, divorce.

III. RISK FACTORS FOR POTENTIALLY VIOLENT SITUATIONS

A. Scenes involving drugs or alcohol

B. Large crowds or violent incidents (domestic disturbances)

C. Patients who are tense, agitated, pacing, aggressive, swearing, yelling, clenching fists

D. Suicidal patients

E. Agitated delirium patients

IV. GENERAL MANAGEMENT OF BEHAVIORAL EMERGENCY PATIENTS

A. Scene safety

1. Request additional resources.

2. Maintain a safe distance.

3. Have an exit plan.

4. Don't block the patient's means of exit.

5. Don't leave the patient alone or leave your partner alone with the patient.

B. Attempt de-escalation techniques.

1. Be empathetic.

2. Respect the patient's personal space.

3. Use neutral tone and body language (no yelling).

4. Don't overreact and ignore challenging questions.

5. Negotiate when possible, but enforce clear boundaries related to safety.

6. Allow silence and time for decisions.

7. Listen carefully, do not interrupt, ask open-ended questions.

8. Do not rush the patient or give ultimatums.

9. Be nonjudgmental and honest.

C. Consider physiological causes, such as hypoglycemia and hypoxia (check SpO_2 and blood glucose when possible).

D. Transport.

Note: Do not rush these calls. They take as long as they take. When in doubt, contact medical control for assistance.

V. SPECIAL SITUATIONS

A. Suicide

1. Suicide facts

    i. A top-10 leading cause of death in the U.S. for ages 10 to 64.

    ii. Second leading cause of death for ages 10 to 14.

    iii. Men attempt suicide two to three times more often than women.

    iv. 40% of transgender individuals have attempted suicide.

    v. Most suicide attempts involve firearms, drugs, and/or alcohol.

    vi. All suicidal gestures should be taken seriously, especially when patients indicate a clear plan and the means to carry it out.

2. Risk factors for suicide

    i. Previous attempts

    ii. History of depression or other mental illness

    iii. Serious illness or chronic pain

      iv.   Legal, financial, or relationship problems

      v.   Substance abuse

      vi.   Childhood trauma

      vii.   Victim or perpetrator of violence

   3. National 988 Suicide & Crisis Lifeline (call or text). See Chapter 2 for additional information.

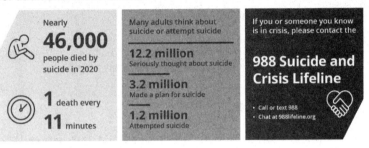

https://www.cdc.gov/suicide/facts/index.html

B. Agitated (excited) delirium

   1. Presentation of agitated delirium

      i.   Acute onset of extreme agitation, aggression, combativeness

      ii.   Hyperactivity

      iii.   Paranoia, panic

   2. Often leads to sudden cardiac arrest. Physical restraint often precedes cardiac arrest.

   3. Typically associated with use of stimulants or hallucinogens (cocaine, methamphetamine, PCP, LSD), psychiatric illness, or head trauma.

   4. Patients frequently exhibit unusual strength, high pain tolerance, and do not tire.

C. Patients exposed to less lethal weapons (Taser conducted electrical weapon, sprays)

   1. Patients that have been tased should be transported once **all** of the following criteria are met:

      i.   GCS of 15.

      ii.   Normal vitals and SpO_2.

      iii. No damage to eyes, face, neck, axilla, groin, breast (females).

      iv. No associated injuries, illnesses, behavioral problems.

      v. Medical direction contacted (per local protocol).

      vi. *Note:* Do **not** remove Taser barbs unless local protocol directs you to do so.

  2. Patients sprayed (pepper spray, etc.)

      i. Patient should be decontaminated before transport.

      ii. Move to area that is ventilated or into fresh air.

      iii. Flush area with water.

      iv. Avoid using soaps.

      v. Remove contaminated clothing.

D. Delirium and dementia

  1. Delirium: acute onset of cognitive problems (confusion, memory loss, dysarthria, hallucinations). Often caused by a treatable medical condition.

  2. Dementia: slow onset of memory impairment. Causes include Alzheimer's disease, AIDS, TBI, Parkinson's disease. Dementia is usually irreversible.

E. Patient restraint (see Chapter 3)

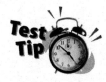
Test Tip

Prepare thoroughly for the national certification exam as quickly as you can. The longer candidates wait, the more the pass rate goes down.

PRACTICE QUESTIONS
Answers on page 395.

1. Which of the following are physiological causes of a behavioral emergency? (Select the TWO answer options that apply.)

    A. anxiety

    B. drugs

    C. paranoia

    D. psychosis

    E. trauma

2. Your patient has been diagnosed with bipolar disorder. This means that the patient experiences

    A. deep, constant sadness.

    B. extreme suspicion of others.

    C. disorganized speech and thinking.

    D. drastic mood swings.

3. Which of the following are known risk factors for suicide? (Select the THREE answer options that apply.)

    A. divorce

    B. promotion

    C. retirement

    D. childhood trauma

    E. previous suicide attempts

    F. thyroid disorders

4. Most suicide attempts involve

    A. jumping from heights.

    B. asphyxiation.

    C. firearms.

    D. hanging.

5. General management of behavioral emergency patients includes

   A. requesting additional resources.

   B. immediately restraining the patient.

   C. demonstrating that you are in charge.

   D. getting the patient alone to talk one on one.

Pediatric and Special Patient Populations

Chapter

28

I. TERMS TO KNOW

A. **Colostomy:** A surgical opening through the abdominal wall.

B. **Fistula:** Surgical connection between an artery and vein for dialysis.

C. **Mottling (mottled):** Abnormal skin color due to vasoconstriction and poor circulation.

D. **Petechiae:** Small, purple spots on the skin.

E. **Stoma:** A surgical opening into the trachea.

> *Note:* Important! Review Chapter 10's special patient situations section regarding pediatric patients.

II. PEDIATRICS

A. Pathophysiology

1. About one in five pediatric deaths is due to injury.

2. Motor vehicle accidents are the leading cause of traumatic injury deaths for children.

3. Respiratory problems are the leading cause of pediatric hospitalizations.

4. Bronchiolitis due to RSV is the leading cause of infant hospitalizations.

B. Anatomy and physiology of pediatrics

1. Airway/respiratory

    i. Tongue: Infants and younger pediatric patients have a proportionally larger tongue than adults. This allows little room for swelling.

    ii. Lower airway: The pediatric lower airway is smaller and more easily obstructed.

    iii. Obligate nose breathers: Most newborns and infants breathe through their nose. Respiratory distress can develop rapidly if the nares are obstructed.

2. Head

    i. The pediatric patient's head is proportionally larger in relation to the body.

    ii. The head is a significant source of heat loss.

    iii. Pediatric patients are at an increased risk of head trauma.

    iv. Sunken fontanelles in infants may indicate dehydration. Bulging fontanelles may indicate increased intracranial pressure.

    v. Children require greater cerebral blood flow. Hypoxia can develop rapidly.

3. Chest/abdomen

    i. Ribs are more pliable, decreasing the risk of rib fractures and increasing the risk of internal injuries.

    ii. Smaller lungs require lower tidal volumes during BVM ventilation. There is an increased risk of lung damage due to overinflation.

    iii. Pediatric patients are often abdominal breathers.

    iv. Abdominal organs are more anterior and less protected.

4. Cardiovascular

    i. Bradycardia should always be viewed as a sign of hypoxia in pediatric patients until proven otherwise.

    ii. Hypotension does not typically develop until the pediatric patient is significantly hypovolemic.

5. Metabolic: pediatric patients typically use oxygen and glucose faster than adults.

6. Skin

    i.   Skin surface area is larger in pediatric patients relative to mass.

    ii. Increased risk of hypothermia.

    iii. Different "rule of nines" for estimating burn surface area (see Chapter 16).

C. Pediatric 9-1-1 calls

   1. Most common pediatric calls are trauma, behavioral, respiratory, seizures, and abdominal pain.

   2. Calls with greatest risk of harm: airway obstruction, respiratory, cardiac arrest, shock, inhalation injury

D. Pediatric assessment triangle (PAT)

   1. Key concepts of PAT

      i. The PAT is intended to be a quick, visual assessment to help determine transport priority.

      ii. You should be able to complete the three key assessments and identify high-priority patients in about 30 seconds.

   2. Appearance (TICLS)

      i.   Tone: assess for movement, muscle tone, listlessness, etc.

      ii. Interactivity: Assess for alertness, reactivity to stimulus, interaction with the environment.

      iii. Consolability: Can the child be consoled by the parents or caregivers?

      iv. Look: Is the child able to fix their gaze, or do they appear "out of it"?

      v.   Speech/Cry: Assess speech in older children or strength of cry in younger children/infants.

   3. Work of breathing: Assess how hard the child is working to breathe, accessory muscle use, lung sounds, grunting, tripod positional breathing, head bobbing, nasal flaring.

    4. Circulation to skin: Assess skin color (e.g., pale, cyanotic, mottled, flushed, jaundice, petechiae).

E. Sudden unexpected infant death (SUID) and sudden infant death syndrome (SIDS)

  1. SUID

    i.   The sudden unexpected death of an infant younger than one year of age.

    ii. Possible causes of SUID include: suffocation, entrapment, infection, airway obstruction, cardiac dysrhythmias, trauma and SIDS.

  2. Sudden infant death syndrome (SIDS)

    i.   SIDS is one form of SUID.

    ii. It is sudden death that cannot be explained even after the autopsy.

F. Child maltreatment

  1. Forms of child maltreatment

    i.   Neglect

    ii. Physical abuse

    iii. Sexual abuse

    iv. Emotional abuse

    v.   Other (abandonment, parental substance abuse, human trafficking)

  2. Signs of maltreatment

    i.   Lack of adult supervision

    ii. Overly compliant, passive, withdrawn

    iii. Caregiver shows lack of concern for the child

    iv. Unexplained injuries, such as burns, bites, bruises, fractures, etc.

    v.   Bruises in various stages of healing

       ➤ Red = less than 24 hours

       ➤ Blue/Purple = 1–4 days

       ➤ Green/Yellow = 5–7 days

       ➤ Disappearing = 1–3 weeks

vi. Shrinks at approach of adults

vii. Explanations that are inconsistent with pattern of injury

viii. Signs of malnutrition

ix. Frequently absent from school

x. Caregiver describes the child negatively or overtly rejects child

3. Shaken baby syndrome/shaken impact syndrome

i. A form of physical abuse that occurs when the infant or child is shaken violently.

ii. Often happens when child won't stop crying.

iii. Can cause permanent brain damage, death.

iv. Signs include irritability, difficulty staying awake, seizures, bruising, vomiting.

4. Burns due to abuse

i. Most burns due to abuse are from hot liquids or other hot objects.

ii. Patterned burns (in clear shape of a hot object) and forced immersion burn patterns are indicative of abuse.

Note: Remember, you are legally required to report suspected abuse to the appropriate authorities.

 III. GERIATRICS

A. Pathophysiology

1. Physiological changes in geriatric patients increase the risk of illness and injury.

i. Cardiac output decreases, blood pressure increases, arteriosclerosis develops.

ii. Lung function is impaired.

iii. Brain shrinks.

iv. Bone mass declines.

2. Falls frequently lead to injury and hospitalization.

B. Communication

1. Speak clearly. Ask one question at a time. Provide additional time to respond.

2. Do **not** assume all elderly patients are hard of hearing or mentally declined.

C. Medical history

1. Nearly 70% of elderly patients have at least two diagnosed medical conditions.

2. Hypertension, heart disease, and diabetes are common.

D. Medications

1. More than half of elderly patients take at least four prescription medications (polypharmacy).

2. Increased risk of medication interactions.

3. Medications are often mismanaged (unsure how to take them, forget to take them, accidentally overdose, or can't afford them).

4. Some medications commonly taken by elderly patients can inhibit the body's ability to compensate for bleeding, shock, or hypotension (e.g., beta blockers, vasodilators, blood thinners, etc.).

E. Environmental cues

1. You are one of the few healthcare providers who will see the patient's living conditions.

2. Is the patient's living situation safe?

3. Signs of abuse, neglect?

4. Does the patient live alone?

5. Does the patient appear equipped to handle tasks of daily living?

F. Specific medical conditions

1. Cardiovascular & respiratory

    i. Myocardial infarction

        ➤ Maintain high index of suspicion for cardiac problems.

        ➤ Geriatric patients often present with atypical signs of MI (see Chapter 12).

    ii. Congestive heart failure

        ➤ Elderly with history of MI or hypertension are at increased risk of CHF (see Chapter 12).

    iii. Pneumonia

        ➤ Elderly at increased risk of pneumonia.

        ➤ Chief complaints of weakness and dyspnea are common.

    iv. Pulmonary embolism: See Chapter 22.

2. Gastrointestinal & musculoskeletal

    i. Elderly patients are at increased risk of GI bleeding and aortic aneurysm (see Chapter 26).

    ii. Maintain high index of suspicion for elderly patients with abdominal pain and hematemesis, hematochezia, melena, coffee ground emesis.

    iii. Osteoporosis is more common in elderly females and often leads to hip and other fractures.

3. Neurological (seizures, stroke, syncope): See Chapter 13.

4. Social/behavioral

    i. Dementia

        ➤ Slow, progressive, irreversible deterioration of cognitive function. Example: Alzheimer's disease.

        ➤ Patients may present with hallucinations, aggressive behavior, limited attention span, diminished motor, social, cognitive abilities.

    ii. Delirium

        ➤ **Unlike** dementia, delirium is a sudden change in cognitive function or mental status.

        ➤ **Unlike** dementia, the causes of delirium can often be treated.

        ➤ Acute anxiety is common; however, memory is often unaffected.

    iii. Depression

        ➤ Depression and suicide rates are high among elderly population.

        ➤ Depression is especially high among patients living in care facilities.

5. Trauma

    i. Increased risk of falls and increased risk of serious injury due to falls.

    ii. Always investigate cause of falls as it may have been preceded by a medical condition (syncope, palpitations, etc.).

IV. SPECIAL PATIENTS

A. At-risk populations include pediatrics, geriatrics, economically disadvantaged, domestic violence victims, and human trafficking victims.

  1. Common presentation in victims of human trafficking

    i. Bruises in various stages of healing

    ii. Scars or infections

    iii. Pelvic pain, rectal trauma

    iv. Pregnancy

    v. Malnourishment, dental problems

    vi. Phobias or panic attacks

  2. Domestic violence victims: Two-thirds of domestic violence victims have injuries to the face, neck, head, or arms.

B. Sensory impairments

  1. Hearing impaired

    i. Face the patient and speak clearly.

    ii. Consider communicating in writing or using closed-ended questions.

    iii. A family member may be able to assist.

  2. Vision impaired

    i. Communicate verbally what you are doing.

    ii. Keep the patient informed about what is happening.

    iii. Protect the patient from injury while moving.

  3. Speech impaired

    i. Ask questions that allow concise answers.

      ii. Allow the patient time to respond and do not finish the patient's statements.

      iii. Do not pretend you understand what the patient is saying if you do not.

C. Developmental disabilities

  1. Most developmental disabilities affect the central nervous system in some way.

  2. Do not assume that a patient's physical appearance is an indication of cognitive dysfunction.

  3. Communicate directly with the patient and keep them informed.

  4. The patient's family and caregivers are likely a valuable resource. Listen to them.

  5. Attempt to determine what the patient's baseline is, and what is different today.

D. Patients with brain injury

  1. Patients with brain injury often rely on extensive medical equipment (ventilators, infusion pumps, feeding tubes, catheters, etc.).

  2. Use caution when manipulating medical equipment. When in doubt, request ALS providers, ask the patient's caregiver, or contact medical control.

  3. Airway and respiratory problems, urinary tract infections, and malnutrition are common.

E. Dialysis patients

  1. Dialysis patients require mechanical assistance to filter toxins from the blood due to poor kidney function.

  2. Patients typically have an implanted device, such as an arteriovenous (AV) shunt, fistula, or graft. These devices connect an artery and a vein to facilitate dialysis.

  3. Do **not** take a blood pressure on an extremity with an AV shunt, fistula, or graft.

  4. Bleeding from AV shunts or fistulas can be severe. Monitor dialysis patients for signs of shock, infection, or bleeding at the site.

  5. Dialysis patients are prone to hypotension and electrolyte imbalances.

V. SPECIAL EQUIPMENT

A. Tracheostomy

1. A tracheostomy is a surgical procedure that creates an opening through the patient's neck into the trachea.

2. A stoma is a surgical opening into the trachea.

3. Patients with a stoma breathe through their stoma, not their mouth or nose.

4. A tracheostomy tube can be placed into the stoma. These tubes can connect to a BVM or a ventilator.

5. Tracheostomy tubes frequently become obstructed by secretions. Be prepared to suction the patient's stoma or tracheostomy tube using a French suction catheter.

6. When providing supplemental oxygen, place the oxygen mask over the stoma.

B. Home ventilators

1. Home ventilators allow automated control of the rate and volume of ventilations and oxygen concentration.

2. Do not manipulate ventilator settings without proper training and medical control authorization.

3. The patient's family and care providers are often familiar with the patient's medical devices, including ventilators.

4. If the patient is not being ventilated adequately, remove the patient from the ventilator and utilize the BVM. Be prepared to suction as needed.

C. Analgesia pumps

1. A patient-controlled analgesia (PCA) pump allows patients to self-administer pain medication through an infusion.

2. The pain medication is typically locked within the PCA and there is a limit to how much medication the patient can self-administer.

3. Follow local protocol regarding management and transport of patients with a PCA.

D. Apnea monitor

    1. Apnea monitors continuously monitor a person's breathing and alarm if breathing stops.

    2. Determine why the patient is on an apnea monitor and how often it alarms.

E. Vascular access device (VAD)

    1. Used for patients who require ongoing venous access for medications, dialysis, chemotherapy.

    2. EMTs do **not** use VADs as a route for medication administration.

    3. Do **not** take a blood pressure on an extremity with a VAD.

F. Feeding tubes

    1. Feeding tubes go from the nose or mouth into the stomach to provide a route for nutrition.

    2. Feeding tubes are used when the patient can't chew or swallow normally.

G. Colostomy

    1. A surgical opening through the abdominal wall allows feces to exit without traveling through the entire GI tract and out the colon.

    2. Patients will typically have a colostomy bag covering the colostomy to collect feces.

    3. Colostomies are prone to infection.

H. Foley catheters

    1. Foley catheters are placed into the urethra and allow urine to drain into a bag.

    2. Patients with an indwelling catheter are prone to infection.

    3. Use extreme caution when moving a patient with a Foley catheter. Keep the catheter positioned low to allow drainage.

I. Intraventricular shunt

    1. An intraventricular shunt allows excess spinal fluid to exit the ventricles of the brain to reduce the risk of increased intracranial pressure (ICP).

2. Intraventricular shunts can become obstructed causing a dangerous increase in ICP.

3. Monitor patients with an intraventricular shunt closely for hypertension, headache, altered mentation, seizures, bradycardia, and respiratory problems.

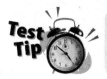

The National EMS Practice Analysis is available through the NREMT. The practice analysis provides information about the most important EMS-related tasks and the current standards for patient care.

PRACTICE QUESTIONS
Answers on page 396.

1. You are assessing a pediatric patient with bradycardia and an altered LOC. Your immediate priority should be

   A. to complete a thorough secondary assessment.

   B. assessment and management of suspected hypoxia.

   C. placement of the AED for further analysis.

   D. administration of oral glucose.

2. What are the key assessments of the Pediatric Assessment Triangle (PAT)? (Select the THREE answer options that apply.)

   A. airway

   B. appearance

   C. BVM ventilation

   D. work of breathing

   E. circulation to skin

   F. check pulse

3. Which of the following statements is correct regarding management of a patient you suspect is being abused?

   A. You are legally required to report suspected abuse to the appropriate authorities.

   B. You can only report suspected abuse to the receiving hospital.

   C. You are not permitted to report suspected abuse without a guardian's consent.

   D. You must have proof of abuse before reporting your suspicions.

4. Your elderly patient complains of abdominal pain, coffee ground emesis, and dark, tarry stool. You should suspect

   A. ingestion of coffee grounds.

   B. stomach flu.

   C. bowel obstruction.

   D. GI bleeding.

5. Your patient is on a home ventilator. The ventilator appears to be malfunctioning. You should immediately

   A. contact medical control for instructions.

   B. try powering off the ventilator and restarting.

   C. begin ventilating the patient with a BVM.

   D. increase the rate and tidal volume of the ventilator.

PART VII

EMS OPERATIONS
REVIEW PLUS
END-OF-CHAPTER PRACTICE

Transport Operations

I. TERMS TO KNOW

A. **Cleaning:** Removing visible contaminants from a surface.

B. **Defensive driving:** Utilization of safe practices for vehicle operations despite surrounding conditions and the actions of others.

C. **Disinfection:** Use of a chemical to kill pathogens.

D. **Sterilization:** Removal of all microbial contamination.

E. **System status management:** Use of data to anticipate demand for EMS and adjust staffing levels and staging locations.

II. GROUND AMBULANCE OPERATIONS

A. Ambulance Design

1. Modern ambulances should meet all the following criteria:

   i. Separate compartments for driver and patient and attendant(s).

   ii. Room for at least two patients and two providers.

   iii. Contain all necessary equipment per local/state requirements.

   iv. Meets state standards for certified ambulance.

   v. Adequate radio communications with dispatchers.

   vi. Capability to establish online medical control.

   vii. Compliance with local, federal, and industry ambulance requirements and safety standards.

   viii. Display a six-point "Star of Life" emblem.

2. Types of ambulances

    i.   Type I: truck cab-chassis with modular ambulance body

    ii.   Type II: standard van design

    iii. Type III: specialty van

    iv. Type IV: heavy duty emergency vehicle

B. Phases of an ambulance call

1. Preparation: Conduct ambulance inspection at start of shift.

2. Dispatch: Determine nature of call, location, number of patients. Notify dispatch you are responding.

3. Travel to scene: Respond safely with due regard.

4. Arrival/patient contact: Position ambulance for safe loading, scene protection/lighting as needed. Notify dispatch you are on scene.

5. Patient transfer to ambulance: Safely transfer and load patient into ambulance. Safely secure patient for transport.

6. Transport to receiving facility: Notify dispatch that you are transporting and to where. Notify receiving hospital per local protocol.

7. Transfer of care: Notify dispatch you have arrived at hospital. Provide verbal report and written PCR. Obtain signature verifying transfer of care.

8. Return to service/post-run: Restock equipment. Clean and disinfect all necessary equipment. Notify dispatch you are back on service.

C. Due regard

1. Emergency vehicle operators can typically disregard most traffic laws when responding in emergency mode (per state laws).

2. Emergency vehicle operators must exercise due regard for safety at all times.

3. Emergency vehicle operators should **never** . . .

    i.   Speed through a school zone.

    ii.   Pass a school bus with the stop sign extended.

    iii. Cross railroad tracks when the warning gates are down.

D. Escorts and multiple-vehicle responses

   1. Police escorts are **not** recommended unless needed for scene safety or if you are lost.

   2. Exercise extreme caution with multiple-vehicle responses, especially at intersections. The likelihood of encountering another emergency vehicle goes up as you get closer to the scene.

E. Defensive driving tactics

   1. Safe arrival is far more important than speed of response. Do **not** sacrifice safety for speed.

   2. Everyone in the emergency vehicle must be properly restrained at all times.

   3. All equipment must be properly secured.

   4. Know your route.

   5. Always know what is next to you in adjacent lanes.

   6. Scan the road frequently.

   7. Keep eyes up while driving.

   8. Maintain safe distance from vehicle in front of you.

   9. Anticipate unexpected actions from other motorists.

   10. Always use daytime running lights.

   11. Always assume other drivers don't see or hear you.

   12. Always assume other drivers will not do what you want them to do.

   13. Always use emergency lights and siren when in emergency mode.

   14. Always stop at red lights and clear intersections.

   15. Always use extra caution at night, at intersections, and during inclement weather.

   16. Avoid "siren syndrome"!

   17. Avoid backing up whenever possible. Always use a spotter.

   18. Pass other vehicles on the left during emergency mode whenever possible.

   19. Know your blind spots.

   20. Minimize distractions while driving.

21. Account for the ambulance's high center of gravity and increased braking distance.

22. Recognize when you are too fatigued to safely operate an emergency vehicle.

F. System status management (SSM)

1. Historic data helps forecast call volume based on time of day and day of week.

2. System status management is used to position ambulances strategically to meet call volume.

3. SSM is data driven; however, it has been widely misused in EMS, contributing to crew fatigue and burnout.

Note: Safety first! During emergency vehicle operations, safety—not speed—is the priority. While the attendant is responsible for patient care during transport, the emergency vehicle operator is responsible for the safety of everyone in the vehicle.

III. AIR AMBULANCE OPERATIONS

A. Types of air ambulances

1. Rotor-wing (helicopter): used for scene calls and local interfacility transport.

2. Fixed-wing (plane/jet): typically used for interfacility transport over about 100 miles.

B. Landing zone (LZ) for rotor-wing aircraft

1. The LZ should be at least 75′ × 75′ during the day and at least 100′ × 100′ at night (follow local protocol).

2. The LZ should be on firm, level ground and clear of overhead obstructions.

3. Keep the LZ clear on approach and departure of the aircraft. The aircraft may return to the LZ unexpectedly if there are mechanical problems.

4. Ensure the LZ is clear of loose debris that could get caught in rotor wash.

5. Do not use tape around the LZ. Do not light LZ with flares, unweighted lights, or blinding strobes.

6. Establish and maintain radio communication with the aircraft during approach, landing, and takeoff.

7. Be prepared to provide the flight crew with basic patient information, patient weight, and destination.

C. Working around EMS helicopters

1. Never approach the aircraft without approval from the pilot.

2. Never approach from the rear of the aircraft.

3. Secure all loose items on the patient, stretcher, and EMS personnel (hats, blankets, etc.).

4. Follow local protocol regarding appropriate use of EMS helicopters and rotor-wing safety.

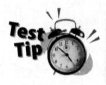

Test Tip

You are likely to see fewer EMS Operations questions on the exam than the other categories; however, you still need to prepare for this category. Make sure you are familiar with the key concepts of the National Incident Management System (NIMS), triage standards, and safety considerations for all types of EMS operations.

PRACTICE QUESTIONS
Answers on page 396.

1. Following a call, you clean and disinfect all the equipment used. This occurs during the

   A. transfer-of-care phase.

   B. post-run phase.

   C. preparation phase.

   D. transport phase.

2. Which of the following are true regarding defensive driving tactics? (Select the THREE answer options that apply.)

    A. The attendant will need to be unrestrained during patient transport.

    B. Keep your eyes on the road directly in front of you.

    C. Anticipate unexpected actions from other motorists.

    D. Pass on the right of other vehicles when possible.

    E. Always use a spotter when backing up.

    F. Driver fatigue is a known hazard to safe vehicle operation.

3. Emergency vehicles are NOT permitted to do which of the following while in emergency response mode?

    A. Speed through a school zone.

    B. Travel above the posted speed limit.

    C. Cross a double yellow line.

    D. Proceed through a red light.

4. You are setting up an LZ for an incoming EMS helicopter. You should

    A. obtain a local weather report and relay it to the pilot.

    B. place a strobe in the center of the LZ.

    C. ensure the LZ is clear of overhead obstructions.

    D. select an LZ that is at least 50' x 50'.

5. When working around an EMS helicopter, you should NEVER approach the aircraft

    A. while it is running.

    B. from the nose.

    C. without a hat on.

    D. from the rear.

Rescue Operations and Hazardous Materials

I. TERMS TO KNOW

A. Complex access: Requires use of special tools and training to access/extricate patient.

B. Entrapment: Being trapped in an enclosed space.

C. Extrication: Removal of a patient from entrapment.

D. Safety data sheet (SDS): Contain detailed information about all hazardous substances on site. Formerly known as material safety data sheet (MSDS).

E. Simple access: Gaining access to the patient without tools or breaking glass.

II. EMS ROLE DURING SPECIAL OPERATIONS

A. Many incidents require personnel with specialized training. Do not attempt operations you have not been trained for.

B. EMS providers' primary role is personal safety and patient care once it is safe to do so.

C. Always wear PPE appropriate for the situation.

D. Rescue operations may include:

1. Vehicle extrication

2. Search and rescue/technical rescue

3. Water rescue

4. Structure fire

5. Law enforcement operations

6. Hazmat incidents

7. Natural disasters

8. MCIs

III. EXTRICATION OPERATIONS

A. Scene safety

1. Leather gloves should be worn over (not instead of) regular PPE gloves when working around glass, sharp objects, rope, etc.

2. Federal law requires use of an approved, highly reflective traffic safety vest when working on roadways, near traffic, or at an accident scene.

B. Vehicle safety systems

1. Shock-absorbing bumpers

   i. Assume all modern vehicles are equipped with shock-absorbing bumpers, front and rear.

   ii. Compressed bumpers can spontaneously release with great force.

   iii. Approach damaged vehicle from sides, not front or rear.

   iv. Do **not** conduct patient care in front of or behind a damaged vehicle.

2. Safety restraint systems (SRS)

   i. Assume all modern vehicles are equipped with multiple SRS airbags (10 or more in some vehicles).

   ii. Airbags deploy at about 200 mph and could be triggered accidentally following an accident (even after battery is disconnected).

      iii. Maintain safe distance (about 2 feet) between you and undeployed airbags.

C. Phases of extrication

  1. Arrival and scene size-up

      i. Position vehicle to improve scene safety.

      ii. Perform 360-degree walk-around if able.

      iii. Determine scene hazards, number of patients, additional resources needed.

  2. Control of hazards

      i. Traffic, fuel leaks, etc.

      ii. Electric and hybrid vehicles

         ➤ *Note:* All orange cables on an electric vehicle are high-voltage; however, **not all** high-voltage cables are orange.

         ➤ Do **not** attempt to disconnect a car battery unless trained to do so.

  3. Patient access

      i. Do **not** attempt to gain access without proper training.

      ii. Keep patient safe while rescuers conduct extrication ops, e.g., blanket, eye protection.

      iii. Rapid extrication is indicated for patients with potentially life-threatening injuries.

Note: Do *not* delay transport of a high-priority patient to manage non-life-threatening conditions.

D. Patient care

  1. Patient care can be performed during extrication ops if safe to do so.

  2. Disentanglement

      i. Simple or complex access (do **not** attempt complex access without proper training and equipment).

      ii. Perform emergency move or urgent move as indicated (see Chapter 3).

3. Patient packaging

    i.   Complete or repeat primary assessment

    ii.   Manage immediate life threats

    iii.   Determine transport priority

    iv.   Complete a thorough patient assessment (high-priority patients should be transported after immediate life threats are managed).

4. Transport to an appropriate facility.

IV. HAZARDOUS MATERIALS

A. The EMT's priorities on a hazmat incident

1. Personal safety

2. Requesting appropriate resources

3. Patient care in a safe zone

B. Hazardous materials training

1. Awareness: Trains responders to recognize potential hazards. Federal law requires all rescue personnel to receive Awareness-level training. (For additional info, visit FEMA: https://training.fema.gov.)

2. Operations: Trains first responders to protect people, property, and the environment. Trained in use of specialized PPE.

3. Technician: Provides significant training related to halting release or spread of hazardous materials.

4. Specialist: Highest level of training. Typically provides assistance at command level.

C. Scene safety considerations

1. Hazardous materials come in many forms. Utilize all your senses to stay alert. When in doubt, get out!

2. All EMS providers should have at least Awareness-level hazmat training.

3. EMS personnel tasks on a hazmat scene include personal safety, notification of appropriate authorities, safety of the public, and patient care in a safe zone.

4. Hazmat resources

   i. Emergency Response Guidebook (ERG)

   ii. Shipping papers

   iii. Safety data sheets

   iv. National Institute for Occupational Safety and Health (NIOSH) Pocket Guide

   v. Police and Emergency Responders' Hazardous Materials Pocket Response Guide

   vi. Wireless Information System for Emergency Responders (WISER)

   vii. Computer-Aided Management of Emergency Operations (CAMEO)

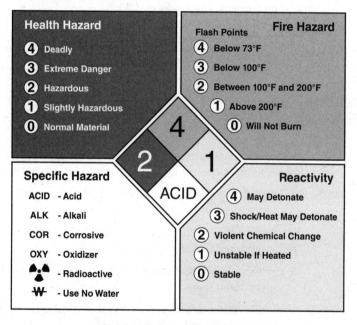

Figure 30-1: Hazmat Warning Placards

D. Emergency Response Guidebook

1. Yellow section: organized by hazardous materials ID numbers.

2. Blue section: organized alphabetically by hazardous materials.

3. Orange section: provides general and specific safety information.

    4. Green section: identifies initial isolation and protective action distances.

E. Placards

    1. Transport of hazardous materials

       i. Vehicles containing hazardous materials in certain quantities are required to display diamond-shaped identification placards.

       ii. Placards contain a four-digit United Nations (UN) identification number. The UN number can be used to identify the hazardous substance.

       iii. All UN numbers listed in ERG prep resources

       iv. Report placard information when requesting additional resources if safe to do so.

    2. Drivers transporting hazardous materials are required to have shipping papers that identify the substance(s) and quantities being shipped.

Note: Always be alert for hazardous materials in non-placarded vehicles (pool cleaners, exterminators, etc.).

    3. Diamond placards used for fixed storage locations with hazardous materials. Placard contains four smaller placards within.

       i. Blue diamond: Provides information about health hazards (numbered 0–4).

       ii. Red diamond: Provides information about fire hazard (numbered 0–4).

       iii. Yellow diamond: Provides information about reactivity hazards (numbered 0–4).

       iv. White diamond: Displays symbols indicating special hazards (radioactivity, reactive to water, etc.).

       v. Numbering: The higher the number, the greater the hazard.

F. Hazmat zones

    1. Hot zone

       i. Contaminated area, requires appropriate PPE.

       ii. Those without proper training and PPE are **not** permitted in the hot zone.

      iii. Patient care does **not** take place in the hot zone.

  2. Warm zone

      i.   Between hot and cold zones.

      ii.   Appropriate PPE required.

      iii. Only life-threatening conditions are treated in warm zone.

      iv. Everyone in warm zone must be decontaminated in warm zone before entering cold zone.

  3. Cold zone

      i.   Most treatment performed in cold zone.

      ii.   Typically, EMS providers remain in cold zone.

G. Decontamination

      i.   Essential to prevent spread of hazardous material.

      ii.   Includes patient's hair, body, clothes, and any medical equipment.

      iii. Decontamination should be performed by personnel trained and equipped to do so.

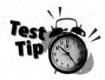

Test Tip

You are almost done with this book! Nice work. To learn more about hazardous materials, visit *https://training.fema.gov*. Look for IS-5.A: Introduction to Hazardous Materials.

PRACTICE QUESTIONS
Answers on page 397.

1. The UN number on a diamond placard is used to

   A. determine the chemical composition of a hazardous material.

   B. identify the hazardous material's origin.

   C. identify the hazardous substance.

   D. determine the quantity of hazardous material being transported.

2. Select the correct statements regarding rescue operations. (Select the TWO answer options that apply.)

   A. Airbags are not a hazard once the vehicle is shut off.

   B. Leather gloves should be worn when working near broken glass.

   C. Compressed bumpers can release spontaneously.

   D. Safety vests are not required during the day.

   E. The safe distance from an undeployed airbag is about 6 inches.

3. What is the EMT's primary responsibility at rescue operations incident?

   A. patient care

   B. assuming incident command

   C. assisting with rescue operations

   D. establishing a treatment section

4. A diamond placard with four smaller placards of different colors is used for

   A. cargo ships.

   B. aircraft.

   C. fixed storage locations.

   D. commercial ground transport vehicles.

5. When working on roadways or around traffic, federal law requires that you

   A. stop traffic in all directions near the incident.

   B. wear an approved, highly reflective safety vest.

   C. wear turnout gear, including helmet.

   D. document the location and condition of all vehicles involved.

Incident Management and Mass Casualty Incidents

I. TERMS TO KNOW

A. **NIMS:** National Incident Management System.

B. **Primary triage:** Takes place early during an MCI, when patients are first encountered.

C. **Secondary triage:** Ongoing triage completed throughout an MCI.

D. **Singular command:** When a single individual has command of the incident. Usually used for single-jurisdiction incidents.

E. **Unified command:** Multiple personnel from different jurisdictions share command.

II. OVERVIEW OF NIMS

A. NIMS priorities are life safety, incident stabilization, and property conservation.

B. NIMS provides an adaptive, standardized approach to any type of domestic incident, e.g., terrorism or natural disaster.

C. NIMS standardizes the command structure, terminology, and training.

D. Standardization improves communication and interaction among multiple and diverse agencies at the local, state, and federal levels.

E. NIMS is adaptable based on size and type of incident.

III. **COMPONENTS OF NIMS**

A. Preparedness: Helps agencies and responders proactively prepare for incidents.

B. Communication and Information: Coordinates effective communication and information sharing.

C. Command and Management: Provides oversight of the incident.

D. Resource Management: Coordinates acquisition, tracking, and recovery of resources and equipment needed during an incident.

 IV. **NIMS PRACTICES**

A. Coordinate efforts through a unified command or single command system to reduce duplication of effort and freelancing.

B. Use "clear text" communication to improve interagency communication and efficiency.

C. Limit span of control to no more than seven workers per supervisor.

 V. **EMS FUNCTIONS OF IMS**

A. Preparedness

1. EMS agencies should have written disaster plans that should be routinely practiced and improved.

2. Plans should include processes to assist families of responders so responders can focus on their duties.

B. Scene size-up

1. Type of incident? Location? Number of patients? Special considerations?

2. First priorities are safety: yourself, your partners/co-workers, patient, and public.

3. Request additional resources as needed.

C. Medical incident command functions

   1. Triage

      i. Triage is the counting and sorting of patients based on severity of injury.

      ii. On large incidents, several responders may be needed to conduct triage.

      iii. On large incidents, patients are moved to treatment areas based on triage status.

      iv. Comprehensive assessment/treatment takes place after all patients are triaged.

   2. Treatment

      i. Patients are moved to established treatment areas.

      ii. Secondary triage conducted in treatment areas.

   3. Transportation

      i. Patients are transported to appropriate destinations without overwhelming receiving facilities.

      ii. Patients typically transported two or more at a time.

   4. Staging: Staging supervisor needed on large incidents to coordinate responding vehicles, agencies, arrival instructions, etc.

   5. Rehabilitation: establishes a safe location for rest and recovery of responders.

   6. Extrication/Special Rescue: established as needed.

VI. TRIAGE METHODS

Note: Determine whether there is a specific triage method in your area. A good understanding of START triage and RAMP triage will prepare you for triage-related questions on the national certification exam.

A. START triage (adults)

   1. Simple Triage and Rapid Treatment (START) developed in Newport Beach, California

2. Four triage categories (see START triage algorithm)

   i.   Immediate (red): highest priority

   ii. Delayed (yellow): second priority

   iii. Minor (green): third priority

   iv. Expectant, aka "dead/dying" (black): fourth priority

3. Uses RPM assessment approach: Respirations, Perfusion, Mental status

4. START triage step 1

   i.   Direct all patients capable of moving to a central location to wait for additional resources.

   ii. Patients capable of moving as directed are considered "Minor," aka "walking wounded" (green tag).

5. START triage step 2

   i.   Begin RPM triage

   ii. Respirations

   ➤ If patient is not breathing, manually open the airway. If patient does not begin breathing, triage as Expectant (black tag).

   ➤ If patient begins breathing when you open the airway, triage as Immediate (red tag).

   ➤ If patient is breathing under 10x/minute or over 30x/minute, triage as Immediate (red tag).

   ➤ If patient is breathing 10–30x/minute, assess perfusion.

   iii. Perfusion (radial pulse)

   ➤ Radial pulse absent: Immediate (red tag)

   ➤ Radial pulse present: assess mental status

   iv. Mental status (simple command)

   ➤ Unable to follow commands: Immediate (red tag)

   ➤ Able to follow commands: Delayed (yellow tag)

B. JumpSTART triage (pediatrics)

   1. Used for patients up to 8 years of age.

2. Similar to START triage, with adaptations for physiological differences in pediatrics

    i. If pediatric patient is apneic with a pulse, provide five rescue breaths.

       ➤ Breathing spontaneously after rescue breaths: Immediate (red tag)

       ➤ No breathing after rescue breaths: Expectant (black tag)

    ii. Breathing below 15x/minute or over 45x/minute: Immediate (red tag)

C. RAMP triage (see RAMP illustration)

1. Rapid Assessment of Mentation and Pulse (RAMP) developed by Rocky Mountain firefighter/paramedic Brad Keating, MPH, NRP.

2. Designed to be faster, easier, more predictive of patient outcomes.

3. Does not require critical thinking, counting respirations or use of triage tags.

4. Works for adult and pediatric patients.

5. Only three triage categories (see illustration).

Figure 31-1: RAMP Triage Model
(Rapid Assessment of Mentation and Pulse)

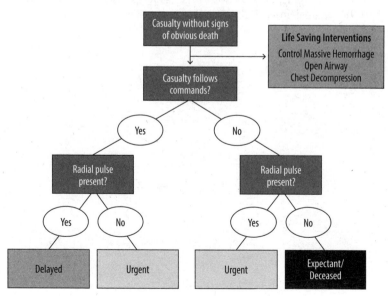

D. Special situations

1. Patients with special needs that cannot be triaged effectively should be moved quickly to treatment area.

2. MCIs involving hazardous materials or terrorism may require additional scene safety precautions before triage can occur.

VII. SPECIAL SITUATIONS

A. Civil unrest

1. May occur during social upheaval, following sporting events, or due to community tension.

2. These events pose higher than normal risk to emergency responders.

B. Tactical Emergency Medical Support (TEMS)

1. EMS specialty involving medical support during military and law enforcement tactical operations.

2. TEMS units deploy and operate in training and high-threat deployments where normal EMS and fire personnel cannot safely respond.

Note: For more information about civil unrest and tactical operations, consult the Fire and Emergency Medical Services Response to Civil Unrest (ems.gov) and the Tactical Emergency Casualty Care (TECC) Guidelines for BLS/ALS medical providers.

PRACTICE QUESTIONS
Answers on page 398.

1. Which of the following provides an adaptive, standardized approach to mass casualty incidents?

   A. NIMS

   B. CISM

   C. SOAP

   D. DNVF

2. During MCIs, radio communications should use

   A. 10 codes approved by the state EMS authority.

   B. encoded digital transmissions only.

   C. clear text communication.

   D. the lead agency's radio codes.

3. Which of the following patients should be triaged as Immediate/Urgent (red)? (Select the TWO answer options that apply.)

   A. A patient who is apneic after opening the airway.

   B. A patient unable to follow commands.

   C. A patient who follows commands and has a weak radial pulse.

   D. An alert pediatric patient breathing 24 times per minute, with a radial pulse.

   E. A patient who follows commands but has absent radial pulses.

4. During an MCI, when does comprehensive patient assessment and care begin?

   A. once all units have arrived on the scene

   B. when the Incident Commander gives the authorization

   C. once all patients have been triaged

   D. following evidence collection

5. When does secondary triage take place?

   A. immediately following primary triage

   B. once ALS personnel arrive on the scene

   C. upon arrival at the hospital

   D. following arrival in the treatment area

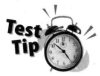

Test Tip

Understand how patients are triaged as **Immediate/Urgent, Delayed,** and **Expectant.** You will almost certainly see triage questions on your national certification exam.

Terrorism and Weapons of Mass Destruction

I. TERMS TO KNOW

A. Biotoxin: Poisonous substance produced by a living organism, such as ricin, botulinum toxin, mold, Lyme, tetanus toxin.

B. CBRNE: Types of weapons (chemical, biological, radiological, nuclear, and explosives).

C. Dirty bomb: Explosive radioactive material in addition to conventional explosives.

D. Pulmonary agent: Chemical agents that irritate or damage the lungs, such as phosgene, chlorine, hydrogen sulfide.

E. Vesicant: Blistering chemical agent, such as mustard gas, lewisite, phosgene oxime.

II. SCENE SAFETY

A. Your safety is your first priority at a terrorism/WMD incident.

B. Follow local protocols and the incident command system (ICS) guidelines.

III. EXPLOSIVES

A. Explosives are the most common WMD.

B. Significant blunt and penetrating trauma are common.

1. Primary blast injuries: caused directly by the blast wave.

2. Secondary blast injuries: caused by flying debris and shrapnel.

3. Tertiary blast injuries: caused by striking the ground or other objects.

4. Quaternary blast injuries: all other explosive-related injuries or disease.

 IV. CHEMICAL AGENTS

A. Many chemicals can be used as weapons without extensive training or financial resources.

B. Nerve agents/organophosphates

1. A significant threat due to the relative ease with which they can be acquired and used.

2. Examples of nerve agents include Tabun, Sarin, Soman, VX.

3. Examples of organophosphates found in over-the-counter pesticides include parathion, diazinon, phosmet, fenitrothion, and more.

4. Nerve agents can cause a massive, life-threatening parasympathetic nervous system response (SLUDGEM). See Chapter 24 for additional information.

5. Anyone with a life-threatening exposure to a nerve agent or organophosphate will likely require atropine and pralidoxime. These two medications are available together in an auto-injector called DuoDote. Consult local protocol regarding EMT administration of atropine or DuoDote auto-injectors.

 V. VESICANTS

A. Vesicants (aka "blistering agents") cause pain, burns, and blisters to exposed skin, eyes, and the respiratory tract.

B. Some vesicants, such as mustard gas, can have delayed onset of symptoms.

C. Irrigate exposed areas continuously with water.

VI. PULMONARY AGENTS

   A. Pulmonary agents (aka "choking agents") cause lung injury.

   B. Signs and symptoms include dyspnea, cough, wheezing, runny nose, sore throat.

   C. Provide oxygen and ventilatory support as needed.

 VII. BIOLOGICAL AGENTS

   A. Used to cause disease.

   B. Even small quantities can cause widespread disease.

   C. Signs and symptoms include fever, weakness, dyspnea, and flu-like symptoms.

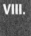 **VIII. NUCLEAR AND RADIOLOGICAL WEAPONS**

   A. Can cause injury and death from the blast, radiation, and thermal burns.

      1. Alpha radiation: Slow-moving radiation that can only travel short distances. Minimal risk due to external exposure, stopped by clothing, skin, etc. Dangerous if inhaled or ingested.

      2. Beta radiation: Can only travel a few feet. Penetrates only the first few millimeters of skin. Serious risk if ingested or inhaled.

      3. Gamma radiation (X-ray): Can travel long distances. Easily penetrates the body. A significant threat to living organisms (all forms of exposure). Signs of radiation sickness include nausea, vomiting, diarrhea, headache, and skin lesions.

      4. Protection from radiation

         i. Time: spend as little time as possible near a radiation source.

         ii. Distance: get as far away as possible from the radiation source.

         iii. Shielding: gamma radiation requires extensive shielding, such as lead or concrete.

Note: To learn more about the EMS aspects of terrorism response and WMD, visit *https://training.fema.gov.* Look for the following online classes: Intro to ICS, Intro to NIMS, Active Shooter, Intro to Hazmat.

PRACTICE QUESTIONS
Answers on page 398.

1. What is the most common weapon of mass destruction?

   A. dirty bomb

   B. biological weapon

   C. conventional explosives

   D. chemical weapons

2. Primary blast injuries are caused by

   A. flying debris and shrapnel.

   B. the blast wave.

   C. striking stationary objects.

   D. penetrating trauma.

3. Which of the following are common symptoms of exposure to a nerve agent? (Select the THREE answer options that apply.)

   A. hyperactivity

   B. salivation

   C. urination

   D. tachycardia

   E. vomiting

   F. pupillary dilation

4. Death due to massive overstimulation of the parasympathetic nervous system is likely caused by which of the following. (Select the TWO answer options that apply.)

   A. mustard gas

   B. phosgene oxime

   C. tabin

   D. gamma radiation

   E. parathion

5. A pulmonary agent is most likely to cause

   A. respiratory distress.

   B. skin lesions.

   C. pupillary constriction.

   D. fever.

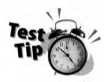

Test Tip

Know the following before taking the national certification exam:

- CBRNE: types of weapons of mass destruction.

- SLUDGEM: nerve agent exposure signs.

- The three protections from radiation (time, distance, shielding).

- The four types of blast injuries.

PART VIII

AFTER THE
EXAM

You Passed. Now What?

Congratulations, you passed the NREMT exam! Welcome to the ranks of the EMS profession. Now what? Here are the author's top 10 recommendations on what you should do next.

ACTION #1: CELEBRATE

Celebrate! You completed an intensive training program and passed a very difficult, comprehensive examination process. You now know better than most that the NREMT only grants EMT certification to those who have earned it. You have demonstrated that you have the knowledge and skills necessary to function competently as a member of the EMS profession. This accomplishment should be celebrated. Take a trip, throw a party, or whatever you do to relax and decompress. Enjoy a break from the rigors of class, homework, tests, etc.

ACTION #2: OBTAIN YOUR STATE LICENSE

Obtain your state EMT license. In most cases, you are not employable as an EMT until you obtain your state license. The process varies from state to state, but is generally quite simple compared to what you have already accomplished. You have most likely already received instructions on how to do this during your EMT course. If not, contact your state EMS authority and ask them how to proceed.

ACTION #3: UPDATE YOUR RÉSUMÉ

Update your résumé. Most professions, including EMS, are moving toward an impersonal, online application process for most jobs. This means that without a good résumé to precede you, you won't likely get a chance to dress sharp, smile, shake hands, or do any of those other things that make a good first impression. Ask your EMT instructor or another local EMS professional to review your résumé and offer suggestions. There are many good résumé templates available online. See the sample résumé at the end of this chapter.

ACTION #4: APPLY YOUR KNOWLEDGE/SKILLS

Get a job! What would you like to do with your EMT certification? You could work on an ambulance or rescue unit. You could work in a hospital emergency department. You could test for the fire department. You could work sporting or concert events. You could join a search and rescue team. There are, most likely, full-time, part-time, and volunteer EMT opportunities within your community. Hopefully, you had a great EMT instructor; however, it's time for experience to be your next teacher. There is no substitute for real-life experience. It's time for you to get some!

ACTION #5: GEAR UP

Determine what equipment is necessary for you to be ready to go to work. For most new EMTs, that should include a good quality stethoscope; a small, high quality tactical flashlight. Last, and most important, ensure you have a strong support system and focus on your own physical and mental health.

Author's Note: Stay safe! Please stay up to date on all of your immunizations, including hepatitis-B and COVID-19.

ACTION #6: JOIN AND READ

EMS is a dynamic profession. This means the one thing you can count on to stay the same is constant change. Find a way to stay engaged in the profession's "big picture." Consider becoming a member of the National Association of EMTs (NAEMT). NAEMT is a respected national organization focused on issues relevant to EMS professionals. Read the "trade journals." The two most widely recognized periodical publications in the EMS profession are the *Journal of Emergency Medical Services* (JEMS) and *EMS World*. Consider subscribing and read them. Both publications include information about job openings around the country and provide access to continuing education opportunities.

ACTION #7: ATTEND AN EMS CONFERENCE

Research the availability of local conferences within your area. This is a great way to earn continuing education credits, and network with fellow EMS professionals, and employers. Most EMS conferences are buffet style, with multiple break-out sessions happening simultaneously. This allows you to pick topics you are most interested in. There are some excellent national EMS conferences, such as the JEMS Conference and Expo, and the EMS World Expo. These annual conferences offer amazing opportunities for learning, networking, and exposure to the latest in EMS equipment, technology, and research.

ACTION #8: BEGIN THE RECERTIFICATION PROCESS

About the time you find out that you passed the certification exam, it's time to start working on your recertification. You have two years before your current national certification expires, but the requirements for recertification are extensive. Don't procrastinate! Visit the NREMT website and become familiar with the recertification requirements. Identify local agencies, hospitals, and educational institutions that offer continuing education opportunities. Research CAPCE-accredited online continuing education opportunities. The NREMT offers some convenient online resources to help track your continuing education and your progress toward meeting the recertification requirements.

Caution: You likely have at least three different expiration dates already. Your CPR certification, state EMT license, and NREMT certification all likely have different expiration dates. Meeting the recertification requirements is your responsibility. Get your expiration dates on your calendar and set reminders to complete recertification requirements on time.

Important: It is **much** easier to maintain your credentials than it is to get them back once they expire.

ACTION #9: DIG DEEPER

Achievement of your credentials should **not** be considered the end of your learning experience. Now you get to pick what you would most like to learn more about. There are additional certifications available in trauma, pediatric emergencies, medical emergencies, newborn resuscitation, hazardous materials, CPR instructor, and much more. Perhaps there are opportunities for you to become a skills tutor or examiner for a local EMT training program. Consider taking an anatomy and physiology class, pathophysiology class, cardiology or pharmacology class, or another subject you're interested in. Ask your EMT instructor what he or she recommends.

ACTION #10: SHOW YOUR GRATITUDE

Thank those that helped you get here. Let your EMT instructor know you passed. Thank your family, friends, employer, coworkers, classmates, mentors, or anyone else that made the journey at least a little easier for you. You will likely lean on some of them again once you decide what the next big challenge will be, like maybe paramedic school!

SAMPLE RÉSUMÉ

[Street Address]
[City, State ZIP Code]
[Telephone]
[Email]

FIRST MIDDLE LAST, NREMT

OBJECTIVE	Employment as an Emergency Medical Technician

SKILLS & ABILITIES	Add something relevant and interesting, such as bilingual

EXPERIENCE	**[JOB TITLE, COMPANY NAME]** [Dates From – To] This is the place for a brief summary of your key responsibilities and most stellar accomplishments.

EDUCATION / CERTIFICATIONS	**ADD COMPLETION OF YOUR EMT COURSE HERE** You might want to include your GPA here and a brief summary of relevant coursework, awards, and honors. **ADD YOUR CPR CERTIFICATION HERE** EX: American Heart Association BLS Healthcare Provider Certification **ADD YOUR STATE EMT CERTIFICATION HERE** EX: EMT certified through the [state] Bureau of Emergency Medical Services. **ADD YOUR NREMT CERTIFICATION HERE** EX: EMT certified through National Registry of Emergency Medical Technicians. **ADD ANY ADDITIONAL CERTIFICATES, DEGREES, ETC. HERE** EX: Online course completion through FEMA Emergency Management Institute.

COMMUNICATION	EX: Strong verbal and written communication skills.

LEADERSHIP	Include leadership experience at work, sports, volunteerism, clubs etc.

REFERENCES	**[REFERENCE NAME]** [Title, Company] [Contact Information]

References

AHA Journals (1999). Should stroke victims routinely receive supplemental oxygen? Retrieved November 27, 2022, from *https://www.ahajournals.org/doi/10.1161/01.STR.30.10.2033*.

AHA Journals (2004). Hyperventilation-induced hypotension during cardiopulmonary resuscitation. Retrieved November 27, 2022, from *https://www.ahajournals.org/doi/10.1161/01.cir.0000126594.79136.61*.

AHA Journals. Optimizing outcomes after out-of-hospital cardiac arrest. Retrieved November 27, 2022, from *https://www.ahajournals.org/doi/10.1161/CIR.0000000000001013#:~:text=The%20use%20of%20AEDs%20increased,3.77%5D%3B%20P%3D0.03*.

AHA Journals. Prognosis of intracerebral hemorrhage related to antithrombotic use. Retrieved November 27, 2022, from *https://www.ahajournals.org/doi/full/10.1161/STROKEAHA.120.030930#:~:text=Intracerebral%20hemorrhage%20(ICH)%20accounts%20for,risk%20of%20death%20and%20disability.&text=The%2030%2Dday%20mortality%20in,patients%20are%20functionally%20independent%20poststroke*.

Alabama Emergency Medical Services and Trauma. BiPAP for prehospital providers. Retrieved November 27, 2022, from *https://www.alabamapublichealth.gov/ems/assets/ems.newsletter081020.pdf*.

American Academy of Orthopedic Surgeons. Human bites. Retrieved November 27, 2022, from *https://orthoinfo.aaos.org/en/diseases--conditions/human-bites#:~:text=Human%20bite%20wounds%20may%20not,caused%20by%20human%20bite%20wounds*.

American Burn Association. Burn center reference criteria. Retrieved November 27, 2022, from *https://ameriburn.org/wp-content/uploads/2017/05/burncenterreferralcriteria.pdf*.

American Heart Association. Hypothermia. Retrieved November 27, 2022, from *https://www.ahajournals.org/doi/10.1161/CIRCULATIONAHA.105.166566*.

American Heart Association (2020). Highlights of the 2020 American Heart Association guidelines for CPR and ECC. Retrieved November 27, 2022, from *https://cpr.heart.org/-/media/cpr-files/cpr-guidelines-files/highlights/hghlghts_2020_ecc_guidelines_english.pdf*.

American Heart Association. AED programs Q&A. Retrieved November 27, 2022, from *https://cpr.heart.org/-/media/cpr-files/training-programs/aed-implementation/aed-programs-qa-ucm501519.pdf*.

American Heart Association (2022). 2015 AHA Guidelines Update for Cardiopulmonary Resuscitation (CPR) and Emergency Cardiovascular Care (ECC) Science. Retrieved November 27, 2022, from *https://professional.heart.org/en/science-news/2015-aha-guidelines-update-for-pr-and-ecc-science*.

American Stroke Association. What is TIA. Retrieved November 27, 2022, from *https://www.stroke.org/en/about-stroke/types-of-stroke/tia-transient-ischemic-attack/what-is-a-tia#:~:text=Approximately%2015%25%20of%20all%20strokes,severe%20stroke%20within%20one%20year*.

Bennett, B. (2017). Bleeding control using hemostatic dressings: lessons learned. Retrieved November 27, 2022, from *https://www.wemjournal.org/article/S1080–6032(16)30287–3/fulltext.*

Botz B, Murphy A. Pelvic binder. Retrieved November 27, 2022, from *https://doi.org/10.53347/rID-85028.*

Cardiac arrest in pregnancy in-hospital ACLS algorithm. Retrieved November 27, 2022, from *https://cpr.heart.org/-/media/CPR-Files/CPR-Guidelines-Files/Algorithms/AlgorithmACLS_CA_in_Pregnancy_InHospital_200612.pdf.*

Centers for Disease Control and Prevention. Venomous spiders. Retrieved November 27, 2022, from*https://www.cdc.gov/niosh/topics/spiders/default.html.*

Centers for Disease Control and Prevention (2022).National diabetes statistics report. Retrieved November 27, 2022, from, *https://www.cdc.gov/diabetes/data/statistics-report/index.html.*

Centers for Disease Control and Prevention (September 2016). Hip fractures among older adults. Retrieved June 3, 2017, from *https://www.cdc.gov/homeandrecreationalsafety/falls/adulthipfx.html.*

Centers for Disease Control and Prevention. Drowning facts. Retrieved November 27, 2022, from *https://www.cdc.gov/drowning/facts/index.html#:~:text=Every%20year%20in%20the%20United,22%20nonfatal%20drownings%20per%20day.*

Centers for Disease Control and Prevention. Facts about traumatic brain injury. Retrieved November 27, 2022, from *https://www.brainline.org/article/facts-about-traumatic-brain-injury#:~:text=Traumatic%20brain%20injury%20(TBI)%20is,30%25%20of%20all%20injury%20deaths.&text=Every%20day%2C%20153%20people%20in,from%20injuries%20that%20include%20TBI.&text=Those%20who%20survive%20a%20TBI,the%20rest%20of%20their%20lives.*

Centers for Disease Control and Prevention. Symptoms of mild TBI and concussion. Retrieved November 27, 2022, from *https://www.cdc.gov/traumaticbraininjury/concussion/symptoms.html.*

Centers for Disease Control and Prevention. Stroke facts. Retrieved November 27, 2022, from *https://www.cdc.gov/stroke/facts.htm#:~:text=About%2087%25%20of%20all%20strokes,to%20the%20brain%20is%20blocked.*

Centers for Disease Control and Prevention (October 2016). Suicide prevention. Retrieved June 3, 2017, from *https://www.cdc.gov/violenceprevention/suicide/index.html.*

Centers for Disease Control and Prevention. Leading causes of death. Retrieved November 27, 2022, from *https://www.cdc.gov/nchs/fastats/leading-causes-of-death.htm.*

Centers for Disease Control and Prevention. Risk and protective factors. Retrieved November 27, 2022 from, *https://www.cdc.gov/suicide/factors/index.html#factors-contribute.*

Center for Suicide Prevention (2012). Women and suicide. Retrieved November 27, 2022, from *https://www.suicideinfo.ca/local_resource/women-and-suicide/.*

Doung, H., Patel, G., Hold, C. (2022). Hypothermia. National Center for Biotechnology Information, U.S. National Library of Medicine. Retrieved November 27, 2022, from *https://www.ncbi.nlm.nih.gov/books/NBK568789/#:~:text=Symptoms%20will%20vary%20based%20on,profound%20(%3C24C)%20hypothermia.*

EMS spinal precautions and the use of the long backboard. Prehospital Emergency Care. July 2013;17(3):392–393.

EMTs Not Allowed to Administer Glucagon. Retrieved from November 27, 2022, from *https://beyondtype1.org/emts-not-allowed-administer-glucagon/.*

Federal Emergency Management Agency, U.S. Department of Homeland Security (May 2017). National Incident Management System. Retrieved June 3, 2017, from *https://www.fema.gov/national-incident-management-system.*

Fernandez, A.R., Studnek, J.R., Margolis, G.S. (2008). Estimating the probability of passing the national paramedic certification examination. *Academic Emergency Medicine* 15:258–264.

Fire and Emergency Medical Services Medical Services Response to Civil Unrest. Retrieved November 28, 2022, from *https://www.ems.gov/pdf/Fire_and_Emergency_Medical_Services_Response_to_Civil_Unrest.pdf.*

Food and Drug Administration. Atropine highlights of prescribing information. Retrieved November 27, 2022, from *https://www.accessdata.fda.gov/drugsatfda_docs/label/2019/212319s002lbl.pdf.*

Fussner, J., Velasco, C. Stroke Coordinator Boot Camp. Retrieved November 27, 2022, from *https://www.heart.org/-/media/files/affiliates/gra/gra-qsi/2019-scbc-presentations/5—assessing-stroke—scores—scales-v2.pdf?la=en.*

Gerber, M. Match supply to demand to provide optimal performance. Retrieved November 27, 2022, from *https://www.ems1.com/leadership/articles/match-supply-to-demand-to-provide-optimal-performance-lCzGI0iT4vinICCY/.*

Hazinski, M., ed. (2010). Highlights of the 2010 American Heart Association guidelines for CPR and ECC. Retrieved June 3, 2017, from *https://www.heart.org/idc/groups/heart-public/@wcm/@ecc/documents/downloadable/ucm_317350.pdf.*

Hettiaratchy, S., Papini, R. (2004). Initial management of a major burn: II—assessment and resuscitation. Retrieved June 3, 2017, from *https://doi.org/10.1136/bmj.329.7457.101.*

Hoffman J, Mower W, Wolfson A, Todd K, Zucker M. Validity of a set of clinical criteria to rule out injury to the cervical spine in patients with blunt trauma. National Emergency X-Radiography Utilization Study Group. The New England Journal of Medicine. July 13, 2000;343(2):94–99.

Hsieh, A. (2011). The basics of CPAP. Retrieved November 27, 2022, from *https://www.ems1.com/ems-products/medical-equipment/airway-management/articles/the-basics-of-cpap-h6Svmf3GjncLTU4c/.*

International Surgery Journal (2019). Epidemiology of acute abdominal pain: a cross-sectional study in a tertiary care hospital of Easter India. Retrieved November 27, 2022, from *https://www.ijsurgery.com/index.php/isj/article/view/3754.*

Johns Hopkins Medicine (2022). Frequently asked questions about eating disorders. Retrieved November 27, 2022 from *www.hopkinsmedicine.org/psychiatry/specialty_areas/eating_disorders/faq.html.*

Johns Hopkins Medicine (2017). Guidelines for assessing orthostatic hypotension should be changed, new study recommends. Retrieved November 27, 2022, from *https://www.hopkinsmedicine.org/news/media/releases/guidelines_for_assessing_orthostatic_hypotension_should_be_changed_new_study_recommends_.*

Johns Hopkins Medicine. Tonic-clonic (grand mal) seizures. Retrieved November 27, 2022, from *https://www.hopkinsmedicine.org/health/conditions-and-diseases/epilepsy/tonic-clonic-grand-mal-seizures.*

Joslin Diabetes (228). EMTs not allowed to administer glucagon. Retrieved November 27, 2022, from *https://www.joslin.org/about/news-media/emts-not-allowed-administer-glucagon.*

Journal of Emergency Medical Services (2007). Patient abandonment: what it is and isn't. Retrieved November 27, 2022, from *www.jems.com/product-announcements/patient-abandonment-what-it-an/#:~:text=In%20EMS%2C%20it%20can%20happen,continuing%20care%20is%20still%20needed.*

Keating, B. RAMP mass casualty triage. Retrieved November 27, 2022, from *http://www. specialoperationsmedicine.org/Documents/2019%20SOMSA/Handouts/THURS-TEMS%20 Keating%20Brad%20RAMP%20triage.pdf.*

Lulla, A., LinLin, T., Hawnwan, P., et al. (2020). The EMS suicide threat. Retrieved November 27, 2022, from *www.hmpgloballearningnetwork.com/site/emsworld/1223779/ce-article-ems-suicide-threat.*

Management of Acute Burn Injuries. JEMS Academy. Retrieved November 27, 2022, from *https://thejemsacademy.com/jems/.*

Mayo Clinic. Subconjunctival hemorrhage. Retrieved November 27, 2022, from *https:// www.mayoclinic.org/diseases-conditions/subconjunctival-hemorrhage/symptoms-causes/ syc-20353826.*

Mayo Clinic. Sickle cell anemia. Retrieved November 27, 2022, from *https://www.mayoclinic. org/diseases-conditions/sickle-cell-anemia/symptoms-causes/syc-20355876.*

Mayo Clinic. Respiratory syncytial virus (RSV). Retrieved November 27, 2022, from *https://www. mayoclinic.org/diseases-conditions/respiratory-syncytial-virus/symptoms-causes/syc-20353098.*

Mayo Clinic. Frostbite. Retrieved November 27, 2022, from *https://www.mayoclinic.org/ diseases-conditions/frostbite/symptoms-causes/syc-20372656.*

Mayo Clinic. Anaphylaxis. Retrieved November 27, 2022, from *https://www.mayoclinic.org/ diseases-conditions/anaphylaxis/symptoms-causes/syc-20351468.*

Mistovich, J., Keith, K. (2010). *Prehospital emergency care*, 9th ed. Upper Saddle River, NJ: Pearson Education.

National Association of EMTs. Guide to building an effective EMS wellness and resilience program (2019). Retrieved November 27, 2022, from *http://www.naemt.org/docs/default-source/ems-preparedness/naemt-resilience-guide-01-15-2019-final.pdf?Status=Temp&sfvrsn=d1 edc892_2.*

National Center for Biotechnology Information, U.S. National Library of Medicine. Epidural hematoma. Retrieved November 27, 2022, from *https://www.ncbi.nlm.nih.gov/books/ NBK518982/.*

National Center for Biotechnology Information, U.S. National Library of Medicine. Aspiration risk. Retrieved November 27, 2022, from *https://www.ncbi.nlm.nih.gov/books/NBK470169/.*

National Center for Biotechnology Information, U.S. National Library of Medicine. Removal of the long spine board from clinical practice: a historical perspective. Retrieved November 27, 2022, from *https://www.ncbi.nlm.nih.gov/pmc/articles/PMC6188081/.*

National Center for Biotechnology Information, U.S. National Library of Medicine. Priapism in acute spinal cord injury. Retrieved November 27, 2022, from *https://pubmed.ncbi.nlm.nih. gov/21647168/.*

National Center for Biotechnology Information, U.S. National Library of Medicine. The effectiveness of junctional tourniquets: a systematic review and meta-analysis. Retrieved November 27, 2022, from *https://pubmed.ncbi.nlm.nih.gov/30507857/.*

National Center for Biotechnology Information, U.S. National Library of Medicine. Mortality from aspiration pneumonia: incidence, trends, and risk factors. Retrieved November 27, 2022, from *https://pubmed.ncbi.nlm.nih.gov/35099619/.*

National Center for Biotechnology Information, U.S. National Library of Medicine. The effectiveness of junctional tourniquets: a systematic review and meta-analysis. Retrieved November 27, 2022, from *https://pubmed.ncbi.nlm.nih.gov/30507857/.*

National Center for Biotechnology Information, U.S. National Library of Medicine. Effect of early pelvic binder use in the emergency management of suspected pelvic trauma: a retrospective cohort study. Retrieved November 27, 2022, from *https://www.ncbi.nlm.nih.gov/pmc/articles/PMC5664718/*.

National Center for Biotechnology Information, U.S. National Library of Medicine. Comparison of hemostatic dressings for superficial wounds using a new spectrophotometric coagulation assay. Retrieved November 27, 2022, from *https://www.ncbi.nlm.nih.gov/pmc/articles/PMC4666077/*.

National Center for Biotechnology Information, U.S. National Library of Medicine. The danger of using pop-off valves for pediatric emergency airway management. Retrieved November 27, 2022, from *https://pubmed.ncbi.nlm.nih.gov/32712036/*.

National Center for Biotechnology Information, U.S. National Library of Medicine. Spinal motion restriction (2021). Retrieved November 27, 2022, from *https://www.ncbi.nlm.nih.gov/books/NBK557714/*.

National Center for Biotechnology Information, U.S. National Library of Medicine. Clinical profile of non-traumatic acute abdominal pain presenting to an adult emergency department. Retrieved November 27, 2022, from *https://www.ncbi.nlm.nih.gov/pmc/articles/PMC4535107/*.

National Center for Biotechnology Information, U.S. National Library of Medicine. Suicidality among transgender youth: elucidating the role of interpersonal risk factors. Retrieved November 27, 2022, from *https://pubmed.ncbi.nlm.nih.gov/32345113/*.

National Center for Biotechnology Information, U.S. National Library of Medicine. It's in the bag: tidal volumes in adult and pediatric bag valve masks. Retrieved November 27, 2022, from *https://www.ncbi.nlm.nih.gov/pmc/articles/PMC7234703/*.

National Center for Biotechnology Information, U.S. National Library of Medicine. Heat emergencies. Retrieved June 3, 2017, from *https://medlineplus.gov/ency/article/000056.htm*.

National Center for Biotechnology Information, U.S. National Library of Medicine. Emergency medical service providers' perception of health-threatening stressors in emergency missions: a qualitative study. Retrieved November 27, 2022, from *https://www.ncbi.nlm.nih.gov/pmc/articles/PMC8365476/*.

National Center for Biotechnology Information, U.S. National Library of Medicine. Ectopic pregnancy. Retrieved November 27, 2022, from *https://www.ncbi.nlm.nih.gov/books/NBK539860/#:~:text=An%20ectopic%20pregnancy%20occurs%20when,not%20recognized%20and%20treated%20promptly*.

National Center for Biotechnology Information, U.S. National Library of Medicine. Anaphylaxis. Retrieved June 3, 2017, from *https://www.ncbi.nlm.nih.gov/pmc/articles/PMC2954079/*.

National Center for Biotechnology Information, U.S. National Library of Medicine. What is a heart attack. Retrieved June 3, 2017, from *https://www.nhlbi.nih.gov/health/health-topics/topics/heartattack*.

National Center for Biotechnology Information, U.S. National Library of Medicine. Traumatic brain injury. Retrieved June 3, 2017, from *https://www.ninds.nih.gov/disorders/all-disorders/traumatic-brain-injury-information-page*.

National Center for Biotechnology Information, U.S. National Library of Medicine. What is deep vein thrombosis. Retrieved June 3, 2017, from *https://www.nhlbi.nih.gov/health/health-topics/topics/dvt*.

National Center for Biotechnology Information, U.S. National Library of Medicine. Suctioning neonates at birth: time to change our approach. Retrieved November 27, 2022, from *https://www.ncbi.nlm.nih.gov/pmc/articles/PMC4139400/*.

National Center for Biotechnology Information, U.S. National Library of Medicine. Supplemental oxygen delivery to suspected stroke patients in pre hospital and emergency department settings. Retrieved November 27, 2022, from *https://www.ncbi.nlm.nih.gov/pmc/articles/ PMC4582959/*.

National Center for Biotechnology Information, U.S. National Library of Medicine. Oxygen supplementation in acute myocardial infarction: to be or not to be? Retrieved November 27, 2022, from *https://www.ncbi.nlm.nih.gov/pmc/articles/PMC4900358/*.

National EMS Scope of Practice Model. Retrieved November 28, 2022, from *https://www.ems. gov/pdf/education/EMS-Education-for-the-Future-A-Systems-Approach/National_EMS_Scope_ Practice_Model.pdf*.

National Implementation of the Model Uniform Core Criteria for Mass Casualty Incident Triage. Retrieved November 28, 2022, from *https://www.ems.gov/pdf/2011/December/10-MUCC_ Options_Paper_Final.pdf*.

National Center for Biotechnology Information, U.S. National Library of Medicine. Prescription drug abuse. Retrieved June 3, 2017, from *https://medlineplus.gov/prescriptiondrugabuse.html*.

National Institute of Child Health and Human Development (2022). Science update: pregnancy-associated homicides on the rise in the United States, suggests NICHD-funded study. Retrieved November 27, 2022, from *https://www.nichd.nih.gov/newsroom/ news/091622-pregnancy-associated-homicide#:~:text=In%202020%2C%20the%20risk%20 of,with%20most%20incidents%20involving%20firearms*.

National Institute of Child Health and Human Development (2017). Sudden Infant Death Syndrome (SIDS). Retrieved November 27, 2022, from *https://www.nichd.nih.gov/health/ topics/sids#:~:text=SIDS%20is%20the%20sudden%2C%20unexplained,reduce%20the%20 risk%20for%20SIDS*.

National Institute of Mental Health. Depression and older adults. Retrieved November 27, 2022, from, *https://www.nia.nih.gov/health/depression-and-older-adults*.

National Registry of Emergency Medical Technicians (n.d.). Cognitive exams general information. Retrieved June 3, 2017, from *https://www.nremt.org/rwd/public/document/ cognitive-exam*.

National Registry of Emergency Medical Technicians (n.d.). Technology enhanced items: sample multiple response items. Retrieved November 27, 2022, from *www.nremt.org/ Document/technologyenhanceditems*.

National Registry's EMS Practice Analysis Accepted for Publication (2021). Retrieved November 28, 2022, from *https://www.nremt.org/News/EMS-practice-analysis-accepted-for-publication#:~:text=National%20Registry%E2%80%99s%20EMS%20Practice%20Analysis%20 Accepted%20For%20Publication,Association%20of%20EMS%20Physicians%E2%80%99%20 journal%2C%20Prehospital%20Emergency%20Care*.

National Registry of Emergency Medical Technicians (2010). 2009 National EMS practice analysis. Columbus, OH: NREMT. National Registry of Emergency Medical Technicians.

National Registry of EMTs' Implementation of the 2015 AHA Guidelines for CPR and Emergency Cardiovascular Care. Retrieved June 3, 2017, from *https://www.nremt.org/rwd/public/ document/news-aha-8-22-16*.

National Registry of EMT's Resource Document on Spinal Motion Restriction/Immobilization. Retrieved November 27, 2022, from *https://www.nremt.org/News/National-Registry-of-EMT-s-Resource-Document-on-Sp*.

Neward, C., Fischer, P., Gestring, M., et al. National guideline for the field triage of injured patients: Recommendations of the national expert panel on field triage, 2021. Journal of Trauma and Acute Care Surgery. Retrieved November 27, 2022, from *https://journals.lww. com/jtrauma/Fulltext/2022/08000/National_guideline_for_the_field_triage_of_injured.19.aspx*.

New England Journal of Medicine (2017). Oxygen therapy in suspected acute myocardial infarction. Retrieved November 27, 2022, from *https://www.nejm.org/doi/full/10.1056/nejmoa1706222.*

Osipoff, J. What you need to know about diabetes in children. Stony Brook University Hospital. Retrieved November 27, 2022, from *https://www.stonybrookmedicine.edu/patientcare/askexpert/diabetesinchildren.*

Pediatric advanced life support (PALS): bradycardia (2018). Retrieved November 27, 2022, from *https://emedicine.medscape.com/article/2066778-overview?reg=1&icd=ssl_login_success_220924.*

Pollak, A., ed. (2021). *Emergency care and transportation of the sick and injured,* 12th ed. Tall Pine Drive, MA: Jones and Bartlett.

Prehospital Emergency Care (2022). Methods and implementation of the 2019 EMS practice analysis. Retrieved November 27, 2022, from *https://www.tandfonline.com/doi/full/10.1080/10903127.2020.1856985.*

Risk Factors of Pulmonary Embolism. Hematology-Oncology Associates of CNY. Retrieved November 27, 2022, from *https://www.hoacny.com/patient-resources/blood-disorders/what-pulmonary-embolism/risk-factors-pulmonary-embolism.*

Roach, M.S. (1992). *The human act of caring.* Ottawa, Ontario: Canadian Hospital Association Press.

Sanders, M., McKenna, K. (2019). *Paramedic Textbook,* 5th ed. Tall Pine Drive, MA: Jones and Bartlett.

Say, S. (2022). 5 things to know about suctioning newborns. Retrieved November 27, 2022, from *https://blog.sscor.com/5-things-to-know-about-suctioning-newborns#:~:text=Routine%20Suctioning%20Is%20Unnecessary,after%20birth%2C%20do%20not%20suction.*

Stiell I, Wells G, Worthington J, et al. The Canadian C-spine rule for radiography in alert and stable trauma patients. JAMA. October 17, 2001; 286(15):1841–1848.

Tactical Emergency Casualty Care (TECC) Guidelines for BLS/ALS Medical Providers. Retrieved November 28, 2022, from *www.c-tecc.org/images/4-2019_TECC_ALS_BLS_Guidelines_.pdf.*

Trauma Facts. New Jersey Human Services. Retrieved November 27, 2022, from *https://www.nj.gov/humanservices/dmhas/initiatives/trauma/Trauma_Facts.pdf.*

U.S. Department of Justice. Burn injuries in child abuse. Retrieved November 27, 2022, from *https://www.ojp.gov/pdffiles/9119016.pdf.*

U.S. Department of Transportation, National Highway Traffic Safety Administration (2009). National emergency medical services education standards. Retrieved June 3, 2017, from *http://www.ems.gov/pdf/811077a.pdf.*

U.S. National Library of Medicine (September 2014). Actidose. Retrieved June 3, 2017, from *https://dailymed.nlm.nih.gov/dailymed/drugInfo.cfm?setid=61801c3a-caf2-4bb7-a56a-dc2ee007eccb.*

What are technology enhanced questions and what do they look like (2019). Retrieved on November 27, 2022 from *What Are Technology Enhanced Questions and What Do They Look Like? | Seeds of Literacy.*

What is Tactical Medicine. American College of Emergency Physicians. Retrieved November 28, 2022, from *https://www.acep.org/tacticalem/about-us/what-is-tactical-medicine/.*

White C, Domeier R, Millin M. EMS spinal precautions and the use of the long backboard—resource document to the position statement of the National Association of EMS Physicians and the American College of Surgeons Committee on Trauma. Prehospital Emergency Care. April 2014;18(2):306–314.

Answer Key and Explanations for End-of-Chapter Practice

CHAPTER 2

1. **A.**

   The EMS White Paper is titled "Accidental Death and Disability: The Neglected Disease of Modern Society."

2. **C.**

   Today's EMS care is based on evidence-based medicine, not what has been done in the past or what others recommend.

3. **B and E.**

   Leadership skills and physical ability are both professional attributes of the EMT. *Note:* This type of multiple-choice question (which requires more than one answer) is called a multiple-response question. You will see such questions on the national certification exam.

4. **A.**

   Strong written and verbal communication skills are roles and responsibilities of the EMT.

5. **D.**

   Transfer of care is one of the five high-risk EMS activities covered in this chapter.

CHAPTER 3

1. A.

This is a scene safety question. Safety is **always** your first priority.

2. B, D, E.

Job stress is unavoidable in EMS. You can develop resiliency skills. Exercise can help reduce stress.

3. C.

CISM is a formal process to help deal with stress.

4. C.

Use a high-efficiency particulate air (HEPA) mask or N95 respirator for suspected airborne disease exposure.

5. B.

Emergency moves are used when the scene is dangerous and the patient must be moved immediately and before providing patient care.

CHAPTER 4

1. C.

This defines scope of practice. It is important to understand the difference between scope of practice and standard of care. "Duty to act" is one of the four components of negligence. There is no "doctrine of certification."

2. A.

This defines standard of care. There is no "EMS expectation clause."

3. C.

Do Not Resuscitate Orders are specific to resuscitation efforts. The other options are much broader than DNRs.

4. **B and C.**

   The four components necessary to prove negligence are: duty to act, breach of duty, damage, and proximate cause.

5. **A.**

   Definitive signs of death include decapitation, decomposition, dependent lividity, and rigor mortis.

CHAPTER 5

1. **D.**

   The FCC oversees radio communications.

2. **C.**

   EMS typically uses clear text communications, not radio codes.

3. **A, E.**

   "Objective" means based on fact, not opinion. B, C, and D are all based on opinion.

4. **A.**

   If you didn't do it, don't say that you did. If you did it, document it.

5. **D.**

   Only use abbreviations approved by your agency and medical director.

CHAPTER 6

1. **D.**

   Movement of air in and out of the lungs (evidenced by chest rise and fall) is called ventilation, or pulmonary ventilation.

2. C.

The frontal plane divides the body into anterior and posterior.

3. B.

From the anatomical position, the lateral bone in the forearm is the radius. The ulna is the medial bone in the forearm.

4. A, D, E.

These are key differences in anatomy between pediatric and adult patients.

5. A.

Inadequate tissue perfusion is called shock, or hypoperfusion. Hypoxia is a lack of oxygen. Anemia is a lack of red blood cells. Hypotension is a low blood pressure.

CHAPTER 7

1. A.

A sunken fontanelle indicates probable dehydration.

2. C.

From birth to one month is a neonate. An infant is up to one year. Toddlers are from one to 3 years old. Preschoolers are from 3 to 6.

3. C.

Separation anxiety is common in younger patients. Allow children to stay with caregivers when possible.

4. A.

Eating disorders are most common in adolescents and young adults up to age 25.

5. C, D.

Physical decline typically begins in middle adulthood. Women usually develop menopause in middle adulthood. Adolescents often do not anticipate the consequences of their actions.

CHAPTER 8

1. B.

Polypharmacy is the simultaneous use of multiple medications by one person.

2. A.

A drop in systolic BP above 20 mmHg or a drop in diastolic BP above 10 mmHg upon standing is called orthostatic hypotension or postural hypotension.

3. C.

A normal blood glucose is between 70 to 140 mg/dL (3.9 to 7.8 mmol/L).

4. A, D.

Pale may indicate poor circulation. Flushed indicates excessive heat, fever, or exertion. Mottling indicates poor circulation.

5. C.

Assess the carotid pulse on children and adults to determine if CPR is indicated. For infants, check the brachial pulse.

CHAPTER 9

1. C.

The purpose of the primary assessment is to identify and manage life-threatening conditions.

2. **A.**

   Unresponsive patients may need CPR, so you must check a pulse immediately.

3. **D.**

   The rapid scan is performed to identify any life-threatening conditions not discovered during the primary assessment.

4. **B, E, F.**

   Level of consciousness and transport priority are part of the primary assessment. Baseline vitals are part of the secondary assessment.

5. **A.**

   The circulation, airway, breathing (CAB) approach is indicated for all unresponsive patients and those with obvious life-threatening external bleeding.

CHAPTER 10

1. **B, C, D.**

   These three assessments are directly related to the patient's respiratory status. Pulses, pupils, and BP are not.

2. **B.**

   Always treat pediatric patients with an ALOC and bradycardia for hypoxia.

3. **C.**

   Oxygen is indicated for any patient with an SpO_2 below 95%. Warm, dry skin and clear bilateral lung sounds are normal findings and do not indicate the need for oxygen. Patients with agonal breathing require BVM ventilation.

4. **A.**

The OPA is contraindicated because the patient is not unresponsive. Suction is not needed because the airway is clear. The airway should be managed with an NPA before determining the need for BVM ventilations.

5. **D.**

Patients with a trach tube breathe through the tube, not their mouth or nose. Supplemental oxygen should be placed over the trach tube.

CHAPTER 11

1. **B, D, F.**

Aspirin and acetaminophen are enteral medications.

2. **A.**

Naloxone (Narcan) reverses the effects of narcotics/opioids.

3. **C.**

Headache and burning under the tongue are common side effects of nitroglycerine, but they are not dangerous.

4. **D.**

EMTs typically do not carry nitroglycerine.

5. **A.**

Activated charcoal is used to reduce absorption of recently ingested toxins.

CHAPTER 12

1. **C, D.**

Unstable angina is unpredictable and is an example of ACS.

2. **A, B, D.**

   JVD and pedal edema typically indicate right heart failure. Pulmonary edema and dyspnea typically indicate left heart failure.

3. **B.**

   Patients on a VAD are typically in heart failure.

4. **C.**

   Two-rescuer infant and child CPR is 15:2.

5. **A.**

   Check a pulse first (CAB) with unresponsive patients to rapidly determine if CPR is indicated.

CHAPTER 13

1. **B.**

   Death to brain tissue due to lack of blood flow is a stroke.

2. **B, D. E.**

   The CPSS has only three assessments; slurred speech, arm drift, facial droop.

3. **A.**

   During generalized seizures, the patient is unresponsive and experiences full-body convulsions.

4. **D.**

   Status epilepticus is a dangerous, life-threatening form of generalized seizures.

5. **A, D.**

   Over age 50 and high blood pressure are both headache "red flags."

CHAPTER 14

1. C.

The head often whips back (hyperextension) during rear-impact collisions.

2. A.

Ejection is most likely with unrestrained occupants in a rollover accident.

3. B.

First collision: car strikes object. Second collision: occupant strikes car. Third collision: internal organs strike interior structures of the body.

4. B, C.

Falls greater than 20 feet (adults) or 10 feet (pediatrics), falls resulting in loss of consciousness, falls in patients over age 65, and falls resulting in shock or multisystem trauma are all high risk.

5. A.

Primary blast injuries are due to the pressure wave of the blast.

CHAPTER 15

1. C.

Shock (hypoperfusion) is inadequate tissue perfusion.

2. A.

The patient's signs and symptoms indicated compensated shock (alert, normal BP).

3. A, D.

Tachycardia and pale, cool, clammy skin are indications of compensated shock. Hypotension, decreased LOC, and irregular breathing are indications of decompensated shock.

4. **C.**

   Pediatric patients vasoconstrict well, so BP can be normal until they near circulatory collapse.

5. **D.**

   If direct pressure is ineffective, a tourniquet should be immediately applied.

CHAPTER 16

1. **A.**

   Circumferential burns go all the way around a body part.

2. **C, D, F.**

   See the Burn Center Referral Criteria.

3. **A.**

   The palm of the patient's hand equals about 1% of the patient's TBSA.

4. **D.**

   Crush injuries can be open or closed.

5. **C.**

   Impaled objects should be removed if they prevent airway management, ventilatory support, or chest compressions.

CHAPTER 17

1. **C.**

   Suspect a limb-threatening injury any time there are indications of poor distal circulation.

2. **A.**

   Ground-level falls are the most common cause of hip fractures in elderly patients.

3. **B, E.**

   Femur and pelvic/hip fractures post the greatest risk of bleeding, pulmonary embolism, and sepsis.

4. **C.**

   Your priority is the patient, not the amputated part. Do not delay transport or place an amputated part on ice.

5. **B.**

   You must immobilize the injured bone(s) and the joints above and below the bones.

CHAPTER 18

1. **B.**

   Battle's sign and raccoon eyes are indications of possible basal skull fracture.

2. **B, C.**

   A rigid collar and the ambulance stretcher are typically used to provide spinal motion restriction. The long spine board is used only for extrication in most cases.

3. **A.**

   Retrograde amnesia is difficulty remembering events prior to the injury. Anterograde amnesia is difficulty remembering events after the injury.

4. **C.**

   Cushing's response is hypertension, bradycardia, and altered respirations. These findings indicate TBI with increased ICP.

5. **C.**

Patients with an epidural hematoma often present with a sudden and brief loss of consciousness followed by progressive deterioration in consciousness.

CHAPTER 19

1. **D.**

Air trapped in the thorax under positive pressure is a tension pneumothorax.

2. **A.**

A sucking chest wound is an open pneumothorax.

3. **A, C, F.**

Beck's triad includes JVD, muffled heart tones, and narrowing pulse pressure.

4. **D.**

The patient presents with a flail chest injury with respiratory compromise. The immediate intervention must be BVM ventilation.

5. **B.**

Kehr's sign, Cullen's sign, and Grey Turner's sign are all indications of possible internal abdominal bleeding.

CHAPTER 20

1. **C.**

Non-penetrating objects on the sclera can typically be removed by irrigation.

2. A.

The patient presents with signs and symptoms of an orbital fracture.

3. C, D.

Stabilize impaled objects in the eye and keep both eyes closed to prevent passive movement of the implanted object.

4. B.

An avulsed tooth should be placed in sterile, saline-soaked gauze for transport.

5. B.

Apply an occlusive dressing to an open neck wound to reduce the risk of air embolism.

CHAPTER 21

1. A, D.

Cold typically causes peripheral vasoconstriction to conserve body heat and slow metabolic rate (in later stages).

2. B, C.

Heat typically causes peripheral vasodilation to shed excess heat and increase metabolic rate.

3. A.

Rewarming a hypothermic patient must be done carefully to avoid an increased risk of ventricular fibrillation.

4. C.

Heat exhaustion is caused by exposure to a warm environment and dehydration.

5. C.

Cooling measures for heat stroke must be rapid and aggressive.

CHAPTER 22

1. D.

COPD is a slow, chronic respiratory disease that damages the alveoli.

2. A.

These are all signs and symptoms of pulmonary embolism. RSV is most common in pediatric patients. CF is often fatal by early adulthood.

3. A, D.

RSV can live on hard surfaces for hours and most children have contracted RSV by age 2. Pediatric patients are at the highest risk from RSV. RSV causes a runny nose and a dry cough.

4. C.

Hyperventilation syndrome is characterized by rapid breathing and is often associated with distraught patients.

5. A, C, F.

Continuous SpO_2 monitoring is indicated for all patients with respiratory distress. Never hyperventilate with a BVM or have the patient breathe into a paper bag. CPAP and bronchodilator medications (albuterol and Atrovent) may be indicated for dyspnea patients. SpO_2 should be maintained at 94% or higher, not 90%.

CHAPTER 23

1. A.

Insulin causes blood glucose levels to decrease as it moves glucose from the bloodstream into the cells.

2. C, D, E.

Polydipsia = increased thirst, polyuria = increased urinary output, polyphagia = increased hunger.

3. **B.**

   A normal non-fasting glucose should be between 70–120 mg/dL.

4. **D.**

   Once the blood glucose level reaches about 200 mg/dL, glucose will spill into the urine. This increases urinary output.

5. **A.**

   Oxygen and transport are recommended for patients experiencing a sickle cell crisis.

CHAPTER 24

1. **A, D, E.**

   Anaphylaxis causes bronchoconstriction, vasodilation, and hypotension.

2. **B.**

   An epi-pen is indicated for anaphylaxis, not a common allergic response.

3. **C.**

   An overdose of sedatives or opioids will likely cause a decreased LOC and respiratory depression.

4. **D.**

   Signs of opioid overdose include decreased LOC, respiratory depression, and pinpoint pupils.

5. **A.**

   Synthetic cathinones ("bath salts") and methamphetamine are stimulants.

CHAPTER 25

1. **B, E.**

   Cardiac workload increases during pregnancy. Signs of shock can be masked during pregnancy. Pregnant patients should **not** be placed supine.

2. **A.**

   Painful vaginal bleeding during the third trimester is a common presentation for patients experiencing abruptio placenta.

3. **A.**

   These are signs and symptoms of preeclampsia or PIH. During eclampsia, the patient will be seizing.

4. **D.**

   Newborns with a heart rate above 60 but less than 100 must be ventilated with a BVM. Chest compressions are indicated for a heart rate below 60. Blow-by oxygen is indicated for newborns with a heart rate above 100 who are cyanotic.

5. **C.**

   Pregnant patients in the later stages of pregnancy should **not** be supine. This will compress the inferior vena cava and cause dizziness, weakness, nausea, syncope, and hypotension.

CHAPTER 26

1. **C.**

   Acute means rapid, unexpected onset.

2. **A, B, F.**

   Hematemesis, coffee-ground emesis, and dark/tarry stool are all indications of possible internal bleeding.

3. A.

Visceral pain is usually dull, diffuse, and difficult to localize.

4. D.

This is a classic presentation for appendicitis, especially since the patient is 17 and has never had any surgeries.

5. D.

Gastroenteritis is an intestinal infection that presents with cramping, nausea, vomiting, and diarrhea.

CHAPTER 27

1. B, E.

Anxiety, paranoia, and psychosis are psychological or social causes.

2. D.

Bipolar disorder can cause unusual shifts in mood, energy, concentration, or activity.

3. A, D, E.

Each of these is a known risk factor for suicide.

4. C.

Most suicides involve firearms, drugs or alcohol.

5. A.

Additional resources are often needed. The other options are **not** general management principles when dealing with a behavioral emergency.

CHAPTER 28

1. B.

Always assess for hypoxia in pediatric patients that are bradycardic.

2. B, D, E.

Appearance, Work of Breathing, and Circulation to Skin are the three components of the PAT.

3. A.

You must report suspected abuse to the appropriate authorities. Notifying the receiving hospital alone is not adequate. You do not need consent or proof to report suspected abuse.

4. D.

These are all signs of possible internal bleeding.

5. C.

If you suspect a ventilator malfunction, start by removing the patient from the ventilator and initiating BVM ventilation.

CHAPTER 29

1. B.

Cleaning, disinfection, and restocking occur during the return-to-service/post-run phase.

2. C, E, F.

The other options are **not** defensive driving tactics.

3. A.

Never speed through a school zone, pass a school bus with the stop sign extended, or cross railroad tracks while the gates are down.

4. C.

The LZ should be clear of overhead obstructions (powerlines, trees, etc.).

5. D.

Never approach a helicopter from the rear.

CHAPTER 30

1. C.

The UN identification number can be used to identify the specific hazardous substance.

2. B, C.

Leather gloves should be worn during extrication operations. Compressed bumpers can release spontaneously. The safe distance from an undeployed airbag is up to 20 inches. Safety vests should always be worn while working near traffic.

3. A.

After personal safety, the EMT's primary responsibility during rescue operations is patient care.

4. C.

The four-diamond placard is used at fixed storage locations.

5. B.

OSHA requires workers to wear an approved, highly reflective safety vest when working on roads or near traffic.

CHAPTER 31

1. A.

These are benchmarks of the NIMS.

2. C.

Radio communications should be clear text.

3. B, E.

Patient A is *Expectant*. Patients C and D are *Delayed*.

4. C.

Comprehensive assessment and treatment begins after all patients have been triaged.

5. D.

Secondary triage takes place upon arrival in the treatment area.

CHAPTER 32

1. C.

Conventional explosives are the most common WMD.

2. B.

Primary blast injuries are caused by the blast wave.

3. B, C, E.

Remember "SLUDGEM."

4. C, E.

Tabin is a nerve agent and parathion is an organophosphate.

5. A.

Pulmonary agents cause dyspnea, cough, wheezing, runny nose, sore throat.

Index

D

E

O

P

Notes

Notes